"Until relatively recently, there has been little to —————— understanding of those living with borderline personality disorder. In their lucid and deeply compassionate book, Blaise Aguirre and Gillian Galen explore how mindfulness—the essential strategy in dialectical behavior therapy, developed by preeminent psychologist Marsha Linehan—can open the doors to genuine healing. This informative and accessible guide includes a rich set of mindfulness exercises and short case studies to bring inner ease, resourcefulness, and freedom. Whether you experience borderline symptomology, have loved ones who struggle with this condition, or are a therapist seeking to enhance your skills, this book will provide you with invaluable support and inspiration."

—Tara Brach, PhD, author of *Radical Acceptance* and *True Refuge*

"Finally, a practical guide for helping individuals improve their BPD symptoms by applying the core DBT skill of mindfulness. Aguirre and Galen have applied mindfulness to borderline personality disorder in a unique and precise way. This is a book many people suffering from BPD can use to improve the quality of their lives."

—Michael Roy, LCSW, founder and executive director of Clearview Women's Center for Borderline Personality Disorder

"Aguirre and Galen have written a lucid, elegant, and practical book. Speaking directly to the individual with borderline personality disorder, they offer accessible explanations and instructions for applying ancient mindfulness practices to current suffering, destructive urges, waves of emotional pain, and endangered relationships—all in the service of building a life worth living. The authors are effective, even ingenious, in showing how to use each of the six core mindfulness skills in dialectical behavior therapy to address each of the painful features of borderline personality disorder, which include feelings of emptiness, identity disturbances, episodes of dissociation and paranoia, and self-hatred. The vignettes are true-to-life, the explanations of neuroscience and Buddhism are understandable, the prescribed practices are immediately useful, and the whole package is presented with a maximum of clarity, a minimum of jargon, and a tone of compassion. I can't wait to prescribe this book to my patients; indeed, I think it has already made me a better teacher!"

—Charles Swenson, MD, associate clinical professor of psychiatry, University of Massachusetts Medical School, with a private practice of psychiatry and psychotherapy in Northampton, MA

"Bringing together dialectical behavior therapy (DBT), biological science, and mindfulness traditions with their own clinical wisdom, Aguirre and Galen offer a comprehensive user's guide for managing the mental anguish associated with borderline personality disorder (BPD). Whether already experienced or brand new to DBT, those recovering from BPD will find their insights and practices invaluable for growing in self-acceptance and effective living. I highly recommend this book to individuals who feel trapped in a life of suffering."

—Seth R. Axelrod, PhD, associate professor in the department of psychiatry, Yale University School of Medicine

"This small gem of a book takes the reader on a quiet, but powerful journey of healing as the practice of mindfulness is systematically applied to the core problem areas of borderline personality disorder. The authors show exactly how one can take a life filled with suicidal thoughts and self-destructive behaviors and change it by applying mindfulness skills to underlying dysregulation of emotions, thoughts, behaviors, relationships, and experiences of self. They do this through clear explanations, step-by-step instructions, and excellent case examples. By the end, one has a deep appreciation of the central role of mindfulness practice in overcoming borderline pathology and building a live worth living. It also offers actual clinical skills to help patients develop mindfulness skills where it counts. This is an invaluable book for sufferers of BPD and for all who work with them."

—Don Ross, MD, medical director of the Retreat at Sheppard Pratt and clinical associate professor of psychiatry at the University of Maryland

"Blaise Aguirre and Gillian Galen's book offers positive coping skills and real inspiration to people working to move beyond the suffering arising from their struggles with BPD. This clear presentation of the practices of mindfulness and loving kindness ties in closely with their work as dialectical behavior therapists, and is a most valuable contribution."

—Sharon Salzberg, author of *Lovingkindness: The Revolutionary Art of Happiness*, and cofounder of the Insight Meditation Society

"*Mindfulness for Borderline Personality Disorder* is an indispensable book for anyone suffering from BPD. Packed with innovative techniques and ancient wisdom, it answers the often-asked question, *how can mindfulness help me with specific BPD symptoms?* Aguirre and Galen have successfully answered this question with an exceptional book full of concrete exercises and personal examples. They teach us how to build the muscle of mindfulness in all areas of our lives, uniting mindfulness skills with practices of compassion, meditation, and self-reflection. I've found this book to be an essential companion to Marsha Linehan's *Skills Training Manual for Treating Borderline Personality Disorder*, complimenting and expanding on the critical foundation of core mindfulness by helping us apply awareness and compassion to ourselves, our relationships, and the world we live in. My copy of *Mindfulness for Borderline Personality Disorder* is already highlighted and dog-eared after only one reading, and I am certain this valuable book will be an enduring resource and inspiration for all those on the path of BPD recovery."

—Kiera Van Gelder, author of *The Buddha and the Borderline*

"Aguirre and Galen use their combined years of experience working with teens and young adults diagnosed with BPD to produce an excellent book for consumers, family members, and professionals. They review various aspects of mindfulness and how it can help individuals diagnosed with BPD reduce their suffering while increasing their capacity for pleasure and joy. The authors provide helpful instructions on how to set up a formal mindfulness practice as well as how to practice mindfulness in daily living. I commend the authors for taking sophisticated content about mindfulness and borderline personality disorder and making it easy to understand and apply."

—Alec Miller, cofounder of Cognitive and Behavioral Consultants of Westchester and Manhattan and professor of clinical psychiatry and behavioral sciences at Montefiore Medical Center/Albert Einstein College of Medicine, Bronx, NY

"Aguirre and Galen have provided an outstanding contribution to those practicing, learning, or teaching mindfulness. Both the concepts and examples equally serve the novice and the expert, making the book a must-have resource for everyone. Every personal, professional, and public library should have this book on its shelf."

—Perry D. Hoffman, PhD, president of the National Education Alliance for Borderline Personality Disorder

mindfulness
for borderline personality disorder

RELIEVE YOUR SUFFERING USING *the* **CORE SKILL** *of* **DIALECTICAL BEHAVIOR THERAPY**

Blaise Aguirre, MD
Gillian Galen, PsyD

New Harbinger Publications, Inc.

Publisher's Note

Distributed in Canada by Raincoast Books

Copyright © 2013 by Blaise Aguirre and Gillian Galen
          New Harbinger Publications, Inc.
          5674 Shattuck Avenue
          Oakland, CA 94609
          www.newharbinger.com

Cover design by Amy Shoup; Text design by Tracy Marie Carlson; Acquired by Jess O'Brien; Edited by Nelda Street

---

Library of Congress Cataloging-in-Publication Data

Aguirre, Blaise A.
  Mindfulness for borderline personality disorder : relieve your suffering using the core skill of dialectical behavior therapy / Blaise Aguirre, MD, and Gillian Galen, PsyD.
    pages cm
  Summary: "Written by Blaise Aguirre--a prominent psychiatrist specializing in the treatment of borderline personality disorder (BPD)--Mindfulness for Borderline Personality Disorder offers a new, mindfulness-based approach to emotion regulation and the common symptoms associated with BPD. The mindfulness treatments outlined in this book are based on the author's highly successful program at Harvard-affiliated McLean Hospital, and are drawn from dialectical behavioral therapy (DBT), a proven-effective treatment for BPD"-- Provided by publisher.
  Includes bibliographical references.
  ISBN 978-1-60882-565-3 (pbk.) -- ISBN 978-1-60882-566-0 (PDF e-book) -- ISBN 978-1-60882-567-7 (ePub) 1. Borderline personality disorder--Treatment. 2. Mindfulness-based cognitive therapy. I. Galen, Gillian. II. Title.
  RC569.5.B67A39 2013
  616.85'852--dc23
                        2012047472

Printed in the United States of America

19   18   17

15   14   13   12   11   10   9

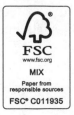

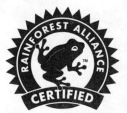

To Lauren, Isabel, Anthony, Lucas, and Gabriel, for, once again, putting up with all the weekends of writing and rewriting.

—Blaise

To Mom, Dad, Barb, and Andy, who taught me gratitude, compassion, and the wisdom in curiosity. To Jed, for honoring and supporting my practice and the many weekends of writing. And to Barbara, my teacher and dear friend, who continues to show me what it means to live mindfully.

—Gillian

Contents

Acknowledgments

Over the years, we have been humbled by our opportunity to work with many people who have struggled with borderline personality disorder (BPD). Before dialectical behavior therapy (DBT) came along, patients with BPD were not always treated with as much compassion or dignity. They were often considered difficult to treat, manipulative, and even undesirable.

We, the professionals—those of us entrusted to care for people with BPD—are to blame for much of the stigma. DBT codified compassion in its "assumptions about patients," stating that those of us who practice DBT will work under the assumption that our patients are doing the best they can; that their lives, as currently being lived, are miserable; and that these people want to change and have lives worth living. We are grateful for the opportunity to be part of the lives of the many people with whom we work, so to the many men and women who have taught us to be mindful, and who shared their stories with us, thank you. To our teachers and colleagues, and, in particular, Michael Hollander, Janna Hobbs, and the staff throughout the years at 3East, thank you. To those who gave us the opportunity to work at McLean and create a dedicated DBT program—Cynthia Kaplan, Joseph Gold, and Phil Levendusky—thank you.

To John Gunderson, who pioneered the early care and treatment of BPD, we thank you and hope that you will join us in the practice of mindfulness one of these days!

To the National Education Alliance for Borderline Personality Disorder (NEABPD), Perry Hoffman, and the many dedicated volunteers working to bring BPD into public awareness, thank you.

To our editorial team at New Harbinger—and, in particular, Jess O'Brien, Jess Beebe, and Nelda Street—who helped us shape the book, and to our agent, Nancy Rosenfeld, who trusted an untested team enough to go through with the proposal, thank you.

Finally, to Marsha Linehan, who started us on the journey all those years ago, thank you.

Introduction

The suffering that underlies the struggle with borderline personality disorder (BPD) is made palpable in these thoughts from Sylvia, a young woman who feels that she has run out of options:

> If life is a long string of painful moments and all you do is die at the end, why can't I just die now? Why does everyone want me to live when my life is so painful? That's why I want to kill myself. I won't do it because it would devastate all the people that I love, but that is why I need your help. I really need to find a way to cope when things are so hard that I just want to give up. I've been trying to stay present just like you suggested but it's so hard. Because wanting to die consumes me so much, I mostly need help finding a reason to live. Some days I can almost see hope. I need your help finding more hope.

If you suffer from BPD, you may be able to relate to Sylvia's struggles.

BPD and Suffering

Using mindfulness to free yourself of the suffering resulting from BPD is a difficult task, in large part because it requires attending to what's going on in your mind. We asked Lauren, a twenty-something-year-old woman with BPD, to consider the difficulties involved in establishing a mindfulness practice. She wrote:

Why the resistance? It is impossible *for me to shut my thoughts off. It only makes me more angry, because I think,* Stop thinking, *and then,* Stop thinking about not thinking, *which leads to* Why is it that I can't not think? *And then I go back to* Here I am, thinking again. *And then I want to hit something, because I'm so frustrated with myself. And even if I were to think about something specific, like* Oh, look how beautiful the trees are, *in the background my brain would think about something else. And then behind all of that, I'd think that my thoughts shouldn't be wandering off and that I need to focus.*

Do you see? Silence is hell. I can't fall asleep without noise, because the noise is the only thing that stops me from thinking. I listen to the TV every single night to fall asleep. If I didn't, I'd never fall asleep. Even as I sit here and write, I'm thinking about the words I'm typing, but I'm also thinking about other things in the background. The more someone tells me not to get caught up in my thoughts, the worse it is—and the more frustrated I get with myself.

A critical breakthrough in the treatment of BPD came with the development of *dialectical behavior therapy* (DBT) by renowned psychologist Marsha Linehan (1993). The explicit application of mindfulness to the treatment presented, for the first time, a way to get people with BPD unstuck from their judgments and intense emotions that lead to suffering. Mindfulness also provides a way to help people who are suffering from BPD to be more effective in applying other useful coping skills in the midst of emotional pain, because mindfulness teaches noticing the emotion without reacting in ways that perpetuate suffering. Through this book, we hope to expand your knowledge and practice of this core DBT skill. We will look at the practice and science of mindfulness, and teach you how to apply it to your BPD symptoms.

Mindfulness and Suffering

For Lauren, the idea of slowing herself down enough to pay attention to her thoughts was intolerable, because it would mean paying attention to all of the pain and suffering in her life. Why would she want to do that? In large part, because research (Chapman, Gratz, and Brown 2006) shows that avoidance of suffering leads to more suffering. Numbing yourself out against the torments of life is a solution, but not a very effective one.

Lauren would rage in the context of feeling misunderstood, particularly during an argument with someone she deeply cared about. Without mindfulness she would say hurtful things and sometimes become self-destructive and suicidal. Her mindfulness practice consisted of noticing her anger and developing the ability to describe her experience: "I'm feeling really angry, hurt, and afraid that you are going to leave me." Recognizing these emotions without acting on them could slow her down enough to allow her to choose her behavior, rather than act mindlessly and make an already miserable situation worse. Rather than say something hurtful, she could use mindful awareness to choose to say or think: "I'm too upset to talk about this right now. I don't want to do something I'll regret later. I need to take some time to get present and out of my head." Such an approach would also mean that she would have time to validate her experience as authentic and understandable, rather than move into behavior that could bring her even more shame and anger.

BPD and Mindfulness

When mindfulness takes hold and the practice is established, suffering begins to melt. Patrick, a young man with BPD, had struggled with various forms of treatment before we introduced to him the idea of mindfulness and how he could begin to get out of his head and pay attention to the reality of the world around him. Desperate to try something new, Patrick threw himself into the practice. After three months he came to a session and said:

I have lived in the same house for twenty years and never noticed just how beautiful my neighbor's garden is. I see so much of my neighborhood that I never realized was there, and people say, "Hi!" I think the mindfulness practices have been helping me a lot, and I know I have a long way to go in terms of really incorporating the techniques into my day-to-day life. I've noticed that my overall anxiety has gone down significantly in the past several months, but it hasn't gone completely. I've become more aware of many of these situations and the impact my anxiety has on my life and my relationship with my girlfriend. I've also noticed that I'm not as depressed as I was over the summer.

We hope that in this book, you will find the wisdom and willingness to practice mindfulness, not only in the moment of struggle, but also as a way of life. And we hope that in so doing, this practice will lead you to the realization that suffering is neither permanent nor inevitable, and, further, that paying attention to things as they are is a path to happiness.

A Quick Guide to This Book

With this book we aim to show you the wisdom and power of mindfulness as a way out of suffering. We have divided the book into four parts.

Part 1 provides you with an overview of borderline personality disorder and of mindfulness. We review the history of BPD and mindfulness, and the ways in which these terms are defined today. Here and throughout the book, we include many stories and insights that people with BPD have shared with us, highlighting their personal struggle and their own introduction to mindfulness.

In part 2 we guide you through the practical application of mindfulness. We expand on this core skill of DBT and introduce a number of other mindfulness practices. You will learn how to develop your own mindfulness practice so that you can use these newly learned skills as a way to take control of your mind and to stop being tossed around by your thoughts and feelings.

In part 3 we explore the lived experience, looking at each symptom of BPD and teaching you specific ways in which you can practice mindfulness to reduce your suffering associated with these symptoms. You will read case vignettes to see how this is done, and you also will learn to recognize the challenges that you may face and to avoid typical pitfalls that you may experience along the way.

In the final part of this book, we look at the journey that awaits you on your mindfulness path. We explore the impact of how you tell the story of your life, and show you how you have the power to change your narrative, particularly when it causes you to suffer.

Making It Useful: Mindfulness Practices

Developing new habits and ways of using your mind can be difficult. To help you develop an understanding of mindfulness and how to use it in your life, we provide illustrative examples throughout the book. We have also highlighted many mindfulness practices. We ask that you bring willingness and an open mind to these practices. Remain curious and take time to observe your experience after doing the practices. Some will be easier than others. Find what works for you.

Remember that the more you practice something, the better you will get at doing it. The exercises in this book are meant to be practiced over and over again, and when you are mindful, you will find that you can repeat practices many times and have different experiences. This book is meant to be a guide to not only teach you about mindfulness, but also teach and support you in an ongoing mindfulness practice.

We hope you find each chapter informative and instructive. If we have accomplished our goal, by the end of this book you will have set foot on a mindful path and feel inspired to continue to practice mindfulness as a way of not only decreasing your suffering from BPD, but also experiencing joy and living your life.

Part 1

Defining Borderline Personality Disorder and Mindfulness

Chapter 1

Borderline Personality Disorder

I f you are like many people who live with borderline personality disorder, you know what it's like to be tossed about by your emotions and to have conflict-ridden relationships with the people you love the most. You may even have experienced self-hatred and how, at times, rage and anger can push loved ones away. You might struggle with the fear that people will abandon you even when they reassure you that they won't. You may know what it is like to feel so miserable that suicide seems like the only way out of your suffering.

It's easy to get discouraged. A moment of intense emotional pain can feel like an eternity. Ask people who don't understand to imagine what ten minutes of a severe toothache feels like—very different from ten minutes of pleasure. Having to suffer through emotional misery on a daily basis leads many people with BPD to think about suicide.

However, the reality is that the vast majority of people with BPD get better, and with the right treatment, many go on to live fulfilling lives. You can join the ranks of the recovered.

You Are Not Alone

Depending on which survey you consult, somewhere between six million and fifteen million people in the United States suffer from BPD (Leichsenring et al. 2011). Sadly, even though BPD is well known to mental health professionals, the general public has barely heard of it. If you are in an outpatient clinic, about 10 percent of your fellow patients will have BPD, and if you end up on an inpatient unit, nearly 25 percent of the other patients will meet criteria for the diagnosis (ibid.).

People often ask about gender differences in BPD. While there is little research on BPD in men, there is growing debate about previous, long-standing data that said that BPD affected women more than men by a ratio of three to one. Research by Bridget Grant and her colleagues (2008) looked at more than thirty-four thousand adults and found that there was no difference in the rate of BPD between men and women. There are a number of theories that try to explain the prior conclusion of a divergence in gender proportions. Some (Giacalone 1997) believe that clinicians have a subtle gender bias toward females with regard to BPD diagnosis, but other research has disputed this. Another possibility (Bjorklund 2006) is that research on the prevalence of BPD is often conducted in psychiatric settings, and because women engage in more self-harming behaviors, there tend to be more women than men with BPD in mental health settings, making it appear that women suffer from this disorder more than men do. So perhaps men with BPD exhibit symptoms like substance abuse or aggressive behaviors that place them in treatment or correctional settings, which are less likely to diagnose BPD. It is our hope that future studies will continue to better define the gender ratios for BPD. At this time, more women than men seek treatment for BPD. So although future research may show that there is an even number of men and women with BPD, in this book you will find more case examples with women than men, in accordance with traditional gender ratios. We hope that all of our readers will use these case examples and not view them as gender specific but, rather, as illustrations of the challenges that all people with BPD can experience.

In the next section, we will examine how BPD is defined.

Defining Borderline Personality Disorder

Since 1938, when many of the recognizable features of modern BPD were first described, the criteria for defining BPD have changed.

Here we will look at how BPD is seen today and then characterize it in a way that will be useful beyond today's definitions. In part 3 of the book we will expand more on the lived experience of BPD and how mindfulness helps to reduce the suffering associated with the symptoms.

BPD and the DSM

The diagnostic criteria for BPD are outlined in the American Psychiatric Association's *Diagnostic and Statistical Manual of Mental Disorders: DSM-IV-TR* (2000), also known as the *DSM*. For a person to be diagnosed with BPD, the *DSM* requires that at least five of nine symptoms be present. One problem with this requirement is that there are 256 possible combinations of symptoms that someone with BPD might experience, which means that you could be in a room with 255 other people struggling with BPD, and each of you could have a different set of symptoms. There are very few, if any, other conditions in medicine where there is so much potential variation. Then, within these 256 possible types, how these people function in life can be very different, so there might be some people with BPD who, despite their difficulties, have stable relationships and are employed or completing their education. Others with BPD have a very difficult time holding on to a job, make repeated suicide attempts, or struggle with impulsivity and have chaotic relationships. For them, visible scars from self-injury and their ways of behaving make it obvious to others that they are struggling with some form of mental illness.

As you can see, there can be tremendous variability in the symptoms that someone with BPD has to deal with. The *DSM* will continue to refine the definition of BPD in updated editions, but regardless, the *DSM* is considered as reflecting the current professional consensus regarding the definition of BPD. You should also know that almost all the professionals making the diagnosis and involved in treatment will use the *DSM* as a reference in their professional training.

The following are the nine *DSM* (2000) criteria for BPD and how they might apply to you.

Efforts to Avoid Abandonment

You might have a strong fear that the people closest to you will abandon you. Jamie, a twenty-seven-year-old with BPD, explained it this way in therapy:

I am unable to be alone, so I do anything to get into a relationship. But then I worry that the person will leave me, so I start to act clingy. The other person doesn't like it when I'm clingy, and begins to push me away. I fear the other person will leave, so I get frantic and then sometimes do bad things to myself, like cutting myself. This freaks out the other person, who then actually does leave, but because I can't stand being alone, I find someone new and the cycle starts all over again.

Your fear of abandonment might be triggered by what seems like a minor rejection, like a friend canceling a plan to go to a movie together or a therapist running two minutes late for an appointment. This fear might lead you to become enraged, because you feel uncared for or unimportant. To others, this rage seems disproportional to the situation at hand, but for you, the suffering and fear are nearly intolerable. When you feel abandoned, you might resort to *reassurance-seeking behaviors*, which are ways of acting that provide reassurance that you will not be left. An example of such behavior is calling or texting your friend or therapist so many times that the person feels annoyed by you. Such behaviors can lead to the destruction of relationships and to the very abandonment that you fear.

Unstable and Intense Interpersonal Relationships

As with the fear of abandonment, you might also recognize the fear of being alone. Often, out of the fear of being alone, some people with BPD tend to attach rapidly and intensely to others in relationships. You might notice the feeling that you have to know whether the other person feels as deeply as you do: that when you love others, they love you as much and that when you suffer, they suffer as much. Because people without BPD don't tend to feel emotions as intensely as you do, they will most likely not respond as deeply as you do, which can feel hurtful. When the hurt is intolerable, you might resort to saying some pretty mean things, simply to get back at the other person. Saying such things can leave you feeling ashamed and regretful about what you said, which may prompt you to swing from delivering demeaning comments to assuring the other person that she is the most wonderful being on earth. For the person you love who is on the receiving end of these extremes of attacks and praise, life gets pretty unpredictable, and often, the person feels that it's too much to handle. These kinds of relationships are stormy and unstable.

Identity Disturbance

Deciding who you are and what your values are can be difficult. You might notice that frequently you have relatively sudden and unexpected changes in your life goals, interests, romantic preferences, and values. These sudden changes can lead to an erratic employment history, wreak havoc in your relationships, and make you unpredictable to others in your life

Impulsivity

When we talk to people who are seeking treatment for BPD, the symptom they say gets them into trouble the most is impulsivity. *Impulsivity* is behaving quickly without evaluating the consequences of the behavior; in fact, sometimes it involves even disregarding potential consequences. In BPD impulsive behavior usually occurs when you have strong emotions or when you are struggling in your relationship. There are many examples of impulsive behavior in BPD, but typically the most dangerous ones are self-injury, drug use, unprotected sex with unknown or casually known partners, and reckless driving. Although these are not necessarily suicidal behaviors, they are dangerous and high-risk behaviors that can seriously affect your long-term health.

Recurrent Suicidal Behavior and Self-Injury

Although suicide is not the same as self-injury, throughout the book we often mention these two behaviors together, because research (Cooper et al. 2005) shows that people who self-injure have an approximately thirty-fold increase in the risk of suicide, compared with the general population. The risk is substantially higher for women who self-injure than for men who self-injure. Suicide rates were highest within the first six months after the first self-harm episode.

So even though suicide and self-injury serve different functions, and it is important to recognize that they are usually behaviors with different goals, they are closely linked.

A total distinction between suicide and what is termed *nonsuicidal self-injury* (NSSI) has been proposed for future editions of the *DSM*. Research shows that whereas many people with BPD self-injure, many others do not, and there are people who engage in NSSI who do not have a personality disorder. Therefore "NSSI disorder" might appear in the next edition of the *DSM*, characterized by high levels of depression, anxiety, suicidality, and poor social functioning (Selby et al. 2012).

Like impulsivity, self-injurious behavior is a common reason why people with BPD seek therapy. As you may have discovered, self-injury works very well to help you regulate your emotions so that you are able to calm down, and few things work as well as cutting. Other reasons why some people with BPD cut themselves are to stop feeling numb and because the physical pain helps distract them from their emotional pain. So you may have discovered a very effective solution for stopping or diminishing your problems, but what you recognize as a solution other people see as a problem. For many parents, friends, and romantic partners, the idea that you cut yourself is very distressing. This distress often pushes the cutting behavior underground. People with BPD tell us that they realize that cutting is not a long-term solution.

With your emotions going up and down, you can feel as if you were being whipped about in the wind, which can make life pretty miserable. Then if your relationships start to fall apart and life becomes particularly miserable, you can begin to wish that you wouldn't wake up some morning or to regard suicide as being the only way out. Usually, thoughts of suicide are just thoughts, but they can be persistent and hard to dislodge from your mind. In some cases the thoughts turn into plans, and the plans turn into suicide attempts. In people with BPD who have been hospitalized, 90 percent will have made at least one suicide attempt and 10 percent will complete suicide (Black et al. 2004). This also means that most suicide attempts are unsuccessful in BPD, and many of these people feel cheated by or ashamed of their failures and attempts. Sometimes people will accuse you of attempting suicide or cutting yourself as a "cry for help" or say that you are "seeking attention." Research shows that these two reasons are rarely the cause of self-injury and suicide (Hollander 2008).

Suicide and Self-Injury: Similar but Different

Earlier we mentioned that there is a close link between suicidal behavior and self-injury, and certainly in BPD, these two behaviors are very closely linked. But as much as they are tied together, they are also separate, and more than 99 percent of all acts of self-injury are done without suicide as a goal. So how do we separate these behaviors in BPD?

Having spent his professional career studying self-injury, Harvard psychologist Matthew Nock has developed a useful way of thinking about these behaviors. Nock (2010) defines self-injury as direct and deliberate bodily harm in the absence of suicidal intent. This definition is useful; however, it is also complicated in that many people with BPD have persistent suicidal thoughts, so teasing the two behaviors apart can be difficult. Therefore, although the following definitions have some overlap and are not distinct categories, we use them in clinical work.

Self-injury. Although self-injury is not classified into different subtypes, Nock and others have suggested that it varies on a scale from mild—which is a low level of severity and frequency—to moderate to severe, which is frequent self-injury that often leads to medical impairment and the need for medical attention.

One question that loved ones often ask us is "Why do people hurt themselves?" Our clinical experience is very similar to the research findings in that most people hurt themselves for one of the following reasons:

- Self-injury relieves their emotional pain.

- It helps them to feel alive or less numb.

- It helps them to focus their attention away from the emotional pain by moving it toward the physical pain.

- It makes someone pay attention to their suffering (this is a rare reason).

- They are addicted to self-injuring and get a rush of energy.

- They feel that they are bad and in need of punishment.

We also see in our clinical work, and others have reported (Strong 1998), that simply thinking or acting on self-injury can reduce suicidal thinking.

There are many other reasons that people give for self-injuring, but these are the most common. As you can see, there is not a mention of suicide in the previous list of reasons for self-harming, so even though many people who self-injure have suicidal thoughts, these behaviors are not one and the same.

Then how do we consider suicidal behavior?

Suicidality. Generally there are considered to be three types of suicidality:

- *Suicidal ideation* means having the thought of killing yourself.

- A *suicide plan* means considering and planning the specific way you would kill yourself.

- A *suicide attempt* means behaving in a potentially self-injurious way in which you have the intention to die.

Emotional Instability

Unstable mood, along with difficulty controlling emotional extremes, is a defining problem for people with BPD. Your mood can shift in a matter of hours. This can be true of people without BPD, but for people with this disorder, the emotional ups and downs are often powerfully triggered by frustration and interpersonal conflict. It is the intensity of the emotions and how uncontrollable they are that makes them different. It is generally believed that people with BPD feel emotions more deeply and for a longer period, and take longer to return to their emotional baseline, than do people who don't have BPD (Linehan 1993). Another aspect is that when you feel a powerful emotion, it can feel to you as if you have always felt that way. So for instance, when you are feeling miserable, you can feel as if you have always been miserable, and you are unable to remember a time when you felt differently, even if just yesterday, you were feeling pretty good. Having other people remind you that your mood state won't last forever hardly seems to help, and can add to the feeling that others don't understand you.

Chronic Feelings of Emptiness

Like many people with BPD, you might experience unrelenting feelings of emptiness. Emptiness is often the feeling of aloneness. This emptiness can lead to difficulties in setting goals and expressing aspirations, which, in turn, can lead to judgment from others that you are uncaring or unmotivated. You might find that being close to others alleviates this sense of emptiness, which makes sense. However, you also run into the problem of others possibly finding your need for closeness to be more than they can provide. So you have to find a balance between being close and being clingy.

Expressions of Intense, Uncontrollable Anger

Mary Jo, a client with BPD who was an assistant manager at a local bookstore, talks about her anger:

I feel like a caged animal pacing back and forth, just wanting out. Everything makes me "frustrated," which is just another word for anger. I'm angry at my boyfriend, who wants to spend more time with his friends than with me; angry at my landlord, who still hasn't fixed the leaky toilet; angry at my boss, who always asks me to cover her shifts; and angry when I hear what my friends are up to, because everyone seems to have a life except for me. Everything seems to make me angry, and you know what I want to do? Smash things and yell. When I was younger, I would smash things, which seemed to help the anger, but now I can't do that.

To others your anger may seem excessive, as if you were making a big deal of small things. You can feel very hurt when people tell you this, which makes you even angrier. Your anger can be something that drives others away.

You can begin to see how all of these symptoms interact with each other. Your anger is difficult for others to tolerate, which causes others to avoid being with you, and then abandonment fears set in.

Paranoid and Dissociative Symptoms

Paranoid thoughts and dissociative symptoms are common in BPD. Typically you would experience these symptoms during times of high stress. You might imagine that other people are intentionally trying to hurt you or make your life miserable. You might experience the feeling that you are not real or that the rest of the world is not real. You might feel disconnected from yourself. These symptoms often appear particularly if there has been abuse or trauma in your life.

BPD and Symptoms Not in the DSM

Although the *DSM* defines the symptoms of BPD, many specific experiences that are typical of living with the disorder are not featured in the *DSM*. You might not experience any of the following symptoms, but many may be familiar to you.

Feeling Misunderstood

You might feel that people don't understand you or why you do the things that you do. This is a common experience in BPD. The truth is that because of the extreme nature of your experiences and emotions, people often don't understand. Not feeling understood often goes together with feeling lonely or alone in the world. Group therapy can be helpful if you have BPD, because you engage with a community of people who share similar experiences.

Self-Hatred

Self-hatred can be another particularly troubling symptom. You might hate how you look. You might feel insignificant, as if you always screw things up and are a terrible person. You might blame yourself for everything bad that happens in your life and the lives of others. You might be quick to dismiss any positive outcome in your life, and come to the conclusion that you are toxic or evil. This thinking can lead to significant self-hatred.

Extreme Sensitivity to Others' Emotions

You may have noticed that you are very sensitive to others' emotions, that when they are anxious, you get all jittery; when they are sad, you get sad; and so on. It might also bother you or seem confusing that others apparently don't pick up on your emotions. And other people might find it unsettling that you can detect what they are feeling even before they do. This can be unsettling to other people in your life who might not be fully aware of their own experiences. In fact, research shows that people with BPD consistently identify others' emotions sooner than do people without BPD (Fertuck et al. 2009). This capacity can lead to trouble when the brief hint of annoyance in the face of a friend triggers an intense fear of abandonment in you. Another tricky situation is when you pick up on happiness in another person and interpret it as intense love rather than joy.

Being "Right" over Being Effective

Almost all of us pride ourselves in the ability to discern right from wrong, and we try to do the "right" thing in any given situation. The idea of what is right can be derived from our faith, our morals, and our values. You might feel that life has not been fair to you and that you must hold on to some position because you are right. This can be problematic, especially when being "right" causes damage to important relationships.

Sarah, who has BPD and is a married mother of a nine-month-old, told us about a fight with her husband:

> We were at a party, and I caught my husband looking at another woman. I know he was looking at her, because she was in good shape and I've put on fifteen pounds over the last year because of my medication. My doctor told me it could happen, but the medication really helps me sleep and controls my moods. I told my husband that night that I was sick of him looking at other women and that I was going to stop taking the medication, because it had made me fat. He told me he loved me, and I said, "If you love me so much, then why do you look at other women?"

He told me he wasn't looking at other women, and it became a huge fight. Anyway I didn't take my medication that night, and I couldn't sleep and was in a foul mood all the next day. I even yelled at my baby. It felt so right not to take my medication.

Sarah felt that a huge injustice had been done and that the right thing to do was to not take her medication. But this caused her to not sleep well and to become more irritable. The effective thing would have been to take the medication even if it didn't feel right. For Sarah, what felt "right" in the moment was driven by her intense emotions.

Lack of a Sense of Continuity of Time

Although you might not experience this symptom, many parents, partners, and clinicians note that people with BPD have difficulty in establishing a continuous and coherent sense of time and sense of self. You might feel that you are living a life of endless repetition, in and out of the same mood states, where you are unable to distinguish one situation from another. This creates the illusion of living a life without time, which can feel intolerable as you imagine that you will never escape. Or you might rapidly get over a long-term relationship as if it had never even happened. This can help you deal with the pain of difficult relationships and emotions. While people may tell you otherwise, you often return to the idea that you have always felt this way. It is as if times of joy, success, or calmness have been eliminated from your memory. If there has been trauma in your life, integrating past events into the present can lead to a fragmented sense of who you are and a feeling that there is nothing of substance there. It can feel as if the pieces and moments of your life don't flow in a straight line, and memories from the past can jump out into the present and feel as if the past events are actually occurring in the present.

Perfectionism

When Claire, a seventeen-year-old high school senior with BPD, was faced with her final essay for English class, she couldn't do it. It was all that stood between her and graduation. Essays had always been difficult, but between her mother's help and her teacher's leniency, she had gotten through. Now she had to write an essay on her own, but she couldn't. She could not imagine a two-thousand-word essay. Paralyzed by the fear that it wouldn't be perfect, she couldn't write a first sentence. Her mother said that Claire had torn up her work after noticing one word out of place.

Perfectionism can show up as extreme obsession about details in your life and work to the point of rigid inflexibility. In the quest for a perfect outcome, you might do and redo a project, and at times never actually get it done. Then you feel overwhelmed by the amount of work that's left to do.

Being Considered Manipulative by Others

Sometimes when we ask people with BPD why they have come into treatment, they say, "To stop being manipulative." When we ask them how they know they are manipulative, they say that others told them they are! Often people with BPD are described as manipulative by clinicians and family members. People in your life will feel manipulated or lied to even if it was never your intention to deceive them or play some trickery. In most situations you might just be doing whatever you can, such as engaging in self-injury to reduce painful emotions. This behavior, however, can feel to others as if you were doing it in order to manipulate or threaten them into doing what you wanted them to do. This is not to say that you are *not* trying to be manipulative, only that just because someone says you are being manipulative doesn't mean that you actually are.

An Integrated Definition of BPD

So, how do you put all of this together? We believe that Marsha Linehan's (1993) approach in reorganizing BPD symptoms into five areas of difficulties, or *dysregulation*, not only is practical, but also will transcend any future editions of the *DSM*. These five areas encompass all of the difficulties outlined in the *DSM*. So the two ways of categorizing BPD are not all that different. For the purposes of this book, we will use Linehan's organization of BPD symptoms as we consider the use of mindfulness for specific symptoms. As we define it, the word "dysregulation" means difficulty in managing—for example, difficulty in managing emotions. Dialectical behavior therapy (DBT) considers five areas of dysregulation in BPD:

Emotion Dysregulation

Emotion dysregulation means that you have difficulty in effectively managing your emotions. You might feel thrown about by your emotions, which are rapidly changing, often in response to conflicts in your relationships. Another aspect of emotion dysregulation is that you might have difficulty with naming, expressing, or fully experiencing emotions.

Interpersonal Dysregulation

Interpersonal dysregulation means that you frequently experience chaos in your relationships, that you have difficulty managing and maintaining your relationships, and that you fear being abandoned by the important people in your life.

Self-Dysregulation

Self-dysregulation means that you have difficulty experiencing yourself as an integrated person, and instead struggle with defining a sense of self. You and others in your life might note that you have changing values, identity, self-image, and preferences. These changes mean that you have trouble developing a good sense of who you are, which can lead to loneliness, boredom, and emptiness.

Behavioral Dysregulation

Behavioral dysregulation means that you use behaviors such as self-injury, suicide attempts, unsafe sex with multiple partners, drug and alcohol abuse, disordered eating, dangerous driving, and other potentially life-threatening behaviors to regulate your emotions.

Cognitive Dysregulation

Cognitive dysregulation means that you might experience episodes of dissociation, where you experience and think about yourself and the world around you as being unreal. You might also experience episodes of paranoia, such as believing that others are intentionally trying to make your life miserable.

BPD as a Skills-Deficit Problem

"My family thinks I intentionally tried to destroy our Thanksgiving weekend," cried Cara, a twenty-eight-year-old nurse with BPD. "I was so excited to see my sister, brother, and parents, but it just wasn't important for them. My sister was with her boyfriend, and my brother didn't want to spend time with me. He just wanted to watch football with my dad, so that left me with my mother. But we still haven't gotten over our last fight, when she told me that my boyfriend was a letch. I felt I was going to explode. It was Thanksgiving. We were supposed to be together. I just started yelling at them that this was supposed to be family time, not TV time or boyfriend time. My mother lost it, and my father yelled at me for being a spoiled brat."

Cara had a hard time waking up that Thursday morning and thought, *I'm going to go to the family house and start yelling at people.* She knew that her family considered her a loose cannon, and she wanted more than anything to be calm, but she was so disappointed that her family didn't like being together that she couldn't contain her sadness and anger.

Like Cara, you might have difficulty controlling your emotions, but this is not because you don't want to but, rather, because you can't. What we mean by this is that although many people are able to control their emotions, emotion regulation is a behavioral skill, like any other skill you might develop. Yelling at someone for never learning to control her emotions is like yelling at someone for never learning to ride a bicycle.

People may think that you have the necessary skills to manage your behavior effectively and yet choose to be obstinate, willful, and angry. We are sure that if the people in your life could see that you are doing the best you can, and could take a more compassionate and nonjudgmental approach to you while you learn the skill of regulating your emotions, life would be easier for you.

Life's Behaviors as Habits

Habits are routines of behavior that are repeated regularly and that occur without your being consciously aware of them. Most of the things you do in your life are habitual in nature and are the product of repetition. Think about the way you brush your teeth, the phrases you use, the way you hold your fork when you eat, the way you respond to people when they talk to you, and so on. Unless you pay very specific attention to the ways in which you do these things, you remain unaware of them and continue to do them habitually.

For most of life's habits, you don't need to pay very close attention, because they are helpful to you in conducting your life. In fact, if you thought about every little thing you did, things would get pretty tedious and interfere with the natural flow of your life. Imagine driving a car and having to think, *Okay, accelerator now, now brake, now clutch, now first gear, now second gear, now indicator, now windshield wipers, now indicator again, now clutch, now third gear, now brake,* and so on. Fortunately you do all of these actions automatically, without conscious thought, because these behaviors have been "hardwired" into your brain and muscles through years of repetition. On the other hand, this hardwiring makes old habits hard to break, which has serious implications for BPD.

How Does Behavior Get Hardwired?

The process of hardwiring any behavior takes place through the frequent repetition of the behavior. These repetitions cause bundles of nerve cells to fire together, which leads to the strengthening of those nerve cells and their neural connections. Think of it as if you were training a muscle. If you train a specific muscle, it becomes stronger, and over time the training becomes easier. If you train yourself in a specific behavior, that, too, becomes easier to do, even if that behavior causes pain and suffering.

Hardwiring Ineffective Habits

In BPD, repeated self-destructive behaviors lead to more of the same; for example, cutting leads to more cutting, repeated suicidal thinking leads to more suicidal thinking, repeated self-hatred leads to more self-hatred, repeated anger leads to more anger, and so on. This is simply the way the brain works. Your brain does not distinguish between playing the piano and cutting with regard to repetition. The more you do it, the better or more efficient you get at doing it. Judgment is what decides that playing the piano is a "good thing" and cutting is a "bad thing." We can rapidly change these judgments through context, so for instance, if a surgeon cuts a person's skin in order to operate, we think of that as a "good thing," and if a person starts playing the piano during a quiet study session in a library, it's a "bad thing." The challenge in BPD is that one habit, such as cutting, may be judged as "bad" by others, whereas for the person with BPD, cutting may be a solution to the problem of intense emotions. To change any repeated behavior, you first must learn to become aware of it, then its context and your judgments about it, and using mindfulness can help.

Effective vs. Ineffective Behavior

Doing what is effective means doing what you have to do to in a specific situation to get a desired goal. If you self-injure in order to relieve emotional pain, self-injury can be effective. However, it usually tends to be effective and helpful only for a short time. It is ineffective as a long-term solution. If it were effective as a long-term solution, you would only have to cut once and be done with it. In this book, as we discuss effective behavior, we mean behavior that helps attain both short-term and long-term goals.

Pathological Certainty

You might find that there are times when you are absolutely certain of other people's thoughts or intentions, and you are incapable of considering any other alternatives. Earlier in this chapter we suggested that it would make your life easier if others cut you some slack and didn't automatically assume that you were intentionally trying to be mean. Similarly, being curious about the motivations behind others' behavior will make your life easier. The reason is that, if you are like many people with BPD, when emotions get the best of you, you assume the worst in others. That can be a very difficult way to live—for instance, believing with certainty that others don't like you. Without any curiosity about how others feel, what their intentions are, or why others behaved in the way they did, you are stuck with assumptions and you believe your assumptions to be real. We call this kind of certainty "pathological," because it leads to suffering and because, in many cases, the assumptions aren't correct.

Cognitive Distortions and All or Nothing Thinking

Cognitive distortions are patterns of thinking in which your brain convinces you that something that isn't true *is* true. Almost every one of us has them. In the case of cognitive distortions, you might tell yourself something that sounds rational but isn't, and your rationalizations can lead to certainty and can perpetuate misery.

There are many different types of distortions. The following are some common ones:

- *Filtering:* This is when you filter out any positive aspects of a situation and dwell just on the negative. You collect data in your mind that confirm the negative aspect of the situation, while ignoring all others pieces of data.

- *Black-and-white thinking:* This is when things are either one way or the exact opposite, and nothing in between, or when the situation cannot have elements of each side within it.

- *Overgeneralization:* This is coming to a broad and general conclusion about something on the basis of a single piece of evidence.

- *Catastrophizing:* This is always expecting or imagining that disaster will occur no matter what, or that terrible things will happen on the basis of a trivial setback.

- *Personalization:* This is when you believe that most of what others are saying, doing, or talking about has to do with you.

- *Fallacy of fairness:* This is when you get resentful because you are certain about what is fair, but others don't agree with you.

- *Belief in "shoulds":* This is when you have rules about the ways in which others *should* behave or the way in which things should be, and then get angry when they aren't that way.

You have learned about the many symptoms of BPD, both the diagnostic criteria and the common symptoms that are not included in the *DSM* but hugely affect the lives of people with BPD. These symptoms can interfere in many areas of your life, and we hope to help you learn ways to develop a mindfulness practice, or expand and add to your current practice in ways that are specific to these symptoms.

In the next chapter we move on to explain what mindfulness is and then follow with examples of how mindfulness can be used to reduce suffering from BPD.

Chapter 2

What Is Mindfulness?

Mindfulness is the core skill of DBT (Linehan 1993). In this book we will take an in-depth look at this core skill and how you can use it as a tool to alleviate the suffering associated with borderline personality disorder. This book will expand your knowledge of mindfulness as it is practiced in DBT, and challenge you to develop this skill more fully. Mindfulness may be unlike anything you have ever done, or the way it is presented in this book may serve to expand your knowledge and practice. Doing something new can be difficult because it's unfamiliar, but keep an open mind. Many people with BPD have found mindfulness to be the way out of their suffering. Before teaching you more about how to use mindfulness, we feel that it's important for you to understand a little about how mindfulness has come to be so central in the treatment of BPD.

Mindfulness Defined

Biologist Jon Kabat-Zinn is a key figure in the research and application of mindfulness in the West. Kabat-Zinn (1994, 4) defines *mindfulness* as "paying attention in a particular way: on purpose, in the present moment, and nonjudgmentally." He believes mindfulness to be fundamental and attainable through practice, and describes it as "a way of being." Others have defined mindfulness as "being present," "staying in this moment," "becoming aware of what's going on around you or within you," and "being in the here and now." For example, you may be mindful of reading this book right now. That is, you are paying attention with an open mind to what you are reading, and when you get distracted by thoughts, feelings, or things going on around you, you purposefully return your attention to the words on the pages of this book. When you bring your attention back, you are being mindful.

Where Did Mindfulness Come From?

The practice of mindfulness, together with the related practice of meditation, has been around for many thousands of years and historically was considered bound to Eastern religion. However, you can find forms of mindfulness and meditation in almost all of the world's religions: there is yogic meditation in the Hindu tradition (Gunaratana 2002), kabbalah meditation in Judaism (Michaelson 2007), contemplative prayer in Christianity (Merton 1960), and Sufi meditation in Islam (Azeemi 2005).

The Eastern Perspective

Each of these religious meditative practices shares the idea of focusing attention. The focus of attention might be on God, on love, on gratitude, on Jesus, on Mohammed, on the heart, or on the breath, but the attention is always focused. For the purposes of this book, we are not looking at mindfulness through the lens of religion, or suggesting that you study Buddhism or become a Buddhist to practice mindfulness. Still, it's important to pay some attention to where this practice originated, and Buddhist philosophy has some important concepts that are quite relevant to the suffering associated with BPD.

Long before modern science, people used their analytical and contemplative abilities along with the power of observation as a way to understand their reality. More than 2,500 years ago, Buddhism noted the idea that we are not static beings, destined to be the same forever. The word "Buddha," translated from the Sanskrit language, means both "to wake up" and "to know." Buddhism recognized that if we "woke up" to the fact that we are changing beings, influenced by our emotions, our biology, and our thoughts, we would not get stuck in thinking that everything, including our misery, will be permanent. People with BPD, all too often, feel that things are never going to change. They feel that they "know" this, but use emotional reasoning as proof. Because of this, they can lose the totality of their experience, by being certain rather than curious, and by not being "awake" to the moment and situation in front of them.

So where does mindfulness fit in? Mindfulness is the English translation of the word *sati* in Pali, the language of Buddhist psychology. Mindfulness is the Buddhist tool that helps people understand their experiences and find freedom from suffering (Gunaratana 2002). It's a practice with roots in the fundamental philosophy, in what are known as "The Four Noble Truths."

The Four Noble Truths

The Four Noble Truths (Tsering 2005) are the central teaching of all Buddhist traditions—Zen, Theravada, Vajrayana—that addresses the concept of suffering and the ability to be still. Keep these ideas in mind, because they will resonate with you as we teach you how to use mindfulness to manage your BPD symptoms. These ideas are considered "noble" because they help us raise our awareness and understanding of all behavior beyond the level of automatic or habitual responses. Developing awareness is a concept that we will return to over and over again in this book.

In the West, we tend to judge suffering as bad and view it as something we must avoid or quickly terminate. Many people with BPD spend much of their lives avoiding pain and suffering through destructive means that often lead to more pain and suffering, so that they never actually find the freedom they are looking for. Buddhism provides a different perspective on the goal of alleviating suffering. We encourage you to come back to these ideas as you reflect on your suffering.

The first noble truth: Life means suffering. Few of us would disagree with this concept, because all of us have suffered, some of us more than others. For many, the suffering can be intolerable. We can feel that it's unfair, and understandably want it to go away. "Life means suffering" simply acknowledges that suffering is a fact of life.

In our lifetimes we will all experience physical pain, such as illness and injury, and psychological pain, such as fear, sadness, disappointment, shame, anger, and depression. All of us will die, and our loved ones will die as well. How do we deal with such suffering? The key here is to remember that nothing is permanent. This can be difficult if you struggle with all-or-nothing, black-and-white thinking (see chapter 1). You will also experience the opposite of suffering, such as joy, comfort, love, calmness, and ease. Suffering is just as much a part of our lives as nonsuffering is. Even though it may not feel like it, our lives are always changing. When you experience joy, it, too, will pass. Joy and suffering flow in and out of our lives all the time. From a Buddhist perspective, suffering is a fundamental part of the human experience and is considered a gift that reminds us of the changing nature of life. But if you are going to change suffering, you must be aware of it in its entirety, not simply how painful it is. This is where mindfulness comes in. While paying attention to suffering can be painful, it is only by paying attention that you can understand suffering and change it (Mruk 2003).

The second noble truth: The origin of suffering is attachment. We will more thoroughly address the concept of attachment in later chapters. Here, the idea is that the origin of suffering is attachment, or holding on to things in our lives, like past hurts, past emotions, past beliefs, and past experiences. Although everything in the past has changed, we can suffer if we hold on to past events as if they were still present today. Often we are not even aware that we are holding on. It's important to remember that we can all fall into the trap of clinging to past hurt, but for people with BPD particularly, such clinging can lead to intolerable pain. To make matters worse, people who suffer from BPD can tend to hold on to past hurt for a very long time.

Any of us can suffer when we expect others to conform to our expectations, when we want to be liked by everyone and aren't, or when we don't get something we want. Getting what we want or expect rarely guarantees long-lasting happiness, and experiencing constant wanting or craving can be an exhausting way to live. Unawareness or lack of understanding of this process leads to suffering and pain; that is, we suffer when we want reality to be different from the way it is. Are there things in your life, such as relationships, goals that are no longer attainable, or anger and resentment, that you find yourself clinging to and that may be causing you distress?

The third noble truth: The cessation of suffering is attainable. Moving on from recognizing that suffering exists, the next idea is that we can overcome suffering and find happiness and peace. With newfound awareness, if we can let go of our craving and clinging, and begin to live in the present—living one day at a time without dwelling in the past or in an imagined future—we can all find greater happiness and free up energy to live our lives more fully. If you are just beginning this journey, you may find this a bit hard to wrap your mind around; however, you will find that mindfulness is the key. If you begin to notice doubt arising within you, remember that mindfulness is challenging, demands practice, and is attainable. There are many people with BPD who have developed advanced mindfulness practices.

The fourth noble truth: There is a path to end suffering. This truth teaches the path to take to end suffering, and it is the path of mindfulness. The foundation of this path is developing awareness of your thoughts and actions, and of compassion for yourself and others. We will teach you to develop this awareness and compassion through the use of mindfulness. As you progress along this path, gain awareness, and practice, the pain of craving and attachment will begin to slowly dissipate.

The Western Perspective

How does this Eastern perspective help? Only in the last few decades has the nonreligious practice of mindfulness become recognized in the West as providing broad benefits to the mind and body. Today, in certain parts of the United States, it is now commonplace to see mindfulness meditation offered throughout communities in schools, clinics, offices, hospitals, and senior centers. Modern scientific techniques, such as brain imaging, are unlocking the secrets of the ancient practice. Mindfulness is now widely studied, and today there are thousands of research papers on the topic. In the late 1970s, Jon Kabat-Zinn formally integrated mindfulness into a therapy by developing Mindfulness-Based Stress Reduction (MBSR). Later he would write (1994, 3):

> Mindfulness is an ancient Buddhist practice, which has profound relevance for our present-day lives. This relevance has nothing to do with Buddhism per se or with becoming a Buddhist, but it has everything to do with waking up and living in harmony with oneself and with the world. It has to do with examining who we are, with questioning our view of the world and our place in it, and with cultivating some appreciation for the fullness of each moment we are alive. Most of all, it has to do with being in touch.

Since the development of MBSR, Kabat-Zinn has found that mindfulness reduces chronic pain (Kabat-Zinn 1982; Kabat-Zinn, Lipworth, and Burney 1985) and symptoms associated with generalized anxiety disorder, panic disorder, and panic disorder with agoraphobia (Kabat-Zinn et al. 1992; Miller, Fletcher, and Kabat-Zinn 1995). Today many researchers have looked at the impact of mindfulness on mood and psychiatric symptoms. For instance, mindfulness practice predicts positive emotional states and improved *self-regulation* (the ability to regulate your own emotions) (Brown and Ryan 2003). Other studies have confirmed that mindfulness practice reduces symptoms of anxiety and depression (Finucane and Mercer 2006; Hofmann et al. 2010), and that it decreases the odds of experiencing a relapse into depression (Teasdale et al. 2000). Additionally, studies have demonstrated improved attention in adults with ADHD (Zylowska et al. 2008), decreased binge eating (Kristeller and Hallett 1999), and decreased post-traumatic stress disorder (PTSD) symptoms of avoidance and numbing in adult survivors of childhood sexual abuse (Kimbrough et al. 2010).

These studies demonstrate the impact of mindfulness on symptoms that many people with BPD struggle with; however, there are fewer studies with participants diagnosed with BPD. A group of researchers in Spain discovered that adding just the mindfulness skills to their general psychiatric treatment improved attention and decreased impulsivity in people with BPD. The researchers also found that the more minutes that the participants practiced mindfulness, the greater the improvement in general psychiatric symptoms and mood symptoms (Soler et al. 2012). A second study found that mindfulness self-observation improved distress tolerance and decreased anger in people with BPD. The authors noted that mindfulness can provide an alternative skill set to rumination when people are angry (Sauer and Baer 2011). A number of empirically validated treatments for BPD, such as dialectical behavior therapy (DBT) (Linehan 1993) and mindfulness-based cognitive therapy (MBCT) (Segal, Williams, and Teasdale 2002), use mindfulness as a core component.

Mindfulness vs. Meditation

You have just read a brief description of mindfulness and how it has become an increasingly accepted practice in Western culture. You have also read how mindfulness has been integrated into medical and psychological treatments. As you learn more about mindfulness, you will likely come across new terminology. We want to clarify some of these new terms. The practice of mindfulness is often discussed with the practice of meditation. Often "mindfulness" and "meditation" are used interchangeably; however, many people consider them to be two distinct yet related ideas. For many people, the idea of meditation conjures up visions of monks isolated in caves or monasteries. In this book we will define *meditation* as a formal way to practice mindfulness. So, if you formally set aside time each day to sit quietly in a certain place and for a certain time, we would define that practice as meditation. Remember that mindful awareness can also be practiced informally (during ordinary daily activities), in which case we would call it "mindfulness," but not "meditation."

Whether through formal meditation or not, our goal is for you to bring awareness through mindfulness into the fabric of your day-to-day life. We will go into the actual practice of mindfulness in much more depth in chapter 4.

Now that you have a sense of what BPD and mindfulness are, we will look at their effects on the brain. In the next chapter, you will begin to see how the neurobiology of mindfulness interacts with the neurobiology of BPD to change the course and nature of BPD.

Chapter 3

The Brain Biology of BPD and Mindfulness

What's a chapter on neurobiology doing in a book on BPD and mindfulness? In chapter 1 you saw that all of the behaviors, thoughts, and emotions that cause you suffering in your struggle with BPD are due to what happens in your brain. For instance, the thoughts *My boyfriend is going to leave me* and *My therapist is going to abandon me* arise in your brain. Your emotional experience flows from your brain. Feeling empty is your brain's interpretation of your current situation. So the "suffering experience" arises in the brain. The good news is that the solution to suffering also arises in the brain. The key is to find more ways to more regularly get your brain to practice and experience joy.

Having a scientific understanding of where in your brain your thoughts and feelings come from means that you can use research findings to focus your therapy on what is causing you to suffer. Think of it this way: Imagine that having a difficult time dealing with your emotions is the same as having a difficult time with walking. Knowing whether your walking difficulty is due to a muscle, bone, or nerve problem would help you decide whether you need to strengthen your muscles, have a broken bone set, or see a neurologist. Troublesome emotions and thoughts are more complicated than a walking problem, but the principle of targeted treatment is the same. The focus should be on what would make your life easier to manage.

The Neurobiology of BPD

The study of brain structure, brain genetics, and brain chemistry, as it applies to behavior, is known as the *neurobiology of behavior*. Neurobiology of behavior looks at looks at how your brain cells organize into circuits and pathways, how these pathways process information, and how all of this leads to behavior. Given how many different types of behaviors there are in BPD, there is no *one* neurobiological explanation for all the symptoms of BPD.

We are often asked if there is a brain scan, blood test, or genetic test that can be used to diagnose BPD. At this time there is no such test; however, there may be brain scans and other tests that, when combined with observable behavior, could be useful in making the diagnosis of BPD.

Studies we'll review later in this chapter will look at how mindfulness can affect the pathways that lead to the behaviors and suffering of BPD. And although mindfulness cannot change your genes, research is beginning to show that it can change the way your genes work (Smalley 2010). Also, although new research emerges on a regular basis about the biology of BPD, we will discuss only the findings that show mindfulness to have an impact.

The Critical Brain Structures

Here is an anatomy lesson to help you better understand the rest of the chapter on BPD and mindfulness. The adult brain weighs about three pounds. The brain connects to the spinal cord through the *brain stem*, which contains bundles of nerve cells, or *neurons*. The largest part of the brain is called the *cerebrum*. The outer layer of the cerebrum is called the *cerebral cortex* (think the skin of an apple), and although it's only a few millimeters thick, it contains nearly one hundred billion nerve cells.

The cerebrum consists of two hemispheres, left and right, and each is divided into four individual *lobes*, known as the *frontal, parietal, temporal,* and *occipital* lobes. Each lobe handles specific behaviors. The frontal lobe deals with decision making, planning actions, and coordinating movements. Just behind the frontal lobe is a region known as the *anterior cingulate cortex*, which regulates heart rate, blood pressure, and breathing rate, and is active during many mindfulness exercises, such as slow breathing.

Deep inside the brain, below each temporal lobe, are the *hippocampus* and the *amygdala*. The hippocampus is primarily responsible for various forms of memory, and we'll describe the role of the amygdala later. The temporal lobe itself contains the part of the brain that deals with hearing as well as processing sound and speech.

In the back of each brain hemisphere is the occipital lobe, which contains the *visual cortex*, where signals from the eyes are processed and interpreted.

We will focus on the two areas of the brain that get the most attention in BPD: the amygdala and the *prefrontal cortex* (PFC). The PFC is located right behind the forehead.

The Amygdala

The amygdala is an almond-shaped group of neurons deep inside each hemisphere of your brain. It processes emotional information. This means that it takes in the emotions that arise in a situation, and allows you to experience the emotions and then decide what to do. The amygdala is most known for managing the *fear response*, which is also known as the *fight-or-flight response*. In people who have BPD, the amygdala is very active, almost too active, so the emotional responses that arise tend to be big. If you have a big emotional response, the behaviors that arise from that response also tend to be big. For example, imagine that your significant other promised to be home by seven and, because of work or traffic, got there fifteen minutes late. You start to get angry as each minute passes, and then by the time he gets home, the anger has boiled over and you blast him. If you were to stand back and think about it, you would likely say that your reaction to his being fifteen minutes late was an overreaction; however, given your powerful emotional response, your behavior seems justified in that moment. In BPD you can blame this response on your overactive, undercontrolled amygdala.

The amygdala also plays an important role in the making of memories—in particular, memories tied to strong emotions. This is a critical function that, under normal circumstances, would work like this: Imagine that you go up to an unfamiliar dog that's wandering in the park, and the dog growls at you and then bites you. You experience fear, and the memory is registered and locked in, making it less likely that you will go up to strange dogs in the future. From an evolutionary perspective, the amygdala would have helped keep us away from all sorts of dangers like saber-toothed tigers. In BPD this response is magnified, and then, rather than their serving simply as a warning system, the memories, paired with strong emotions, play over and over, causing suffering even after the danger has passed, as in the following case:

> When Kathleen, a very sensitive seventeen-year-old with BPD, came to therapy, she seemed engaged and chatty, but whenever her mother came to the therapy session, Kathleen refused to talk. In individual sessions she expressed deep love for her mother, so her behavior when her mother was in the room was confusing. Her mother said that she and Kathleen had been extremely close until Kathleen had turned fourteen. That was when Kathleen's mother had lost her own mother to cancer. She noted that Kathleen had been close to her grandmother but had appeared to have dealt with her grandmother's death as well as could be expected. In therapy Kathleen was working on being able to experience and tolerate her emotions without becoming self-destructive.
>
> One day in therapy, we wondered about her mother's idea that Kathleen's problems had started around the time of her grandmother's death and how before then, Kathleen and her mother had been very close. She agreed that she and her mother had been close.
>
> "Then what happened?"

"When my grandmother died," she said, "I went to my mother and gave her a hug. My mother was crying and was so sad. As she was crying, she talked about her mother and about how empty she felt, that she had lost everything and that now she had no one." Kathleen said that when she heard her mother say that she had no one, she felt more hurt than ever. How could her mother feel that she had no one? She had *her*, Kathleen. How could she possibly say something like that? They had been so close.

Whenever Kathleen saw her mother cry, it would trigger the memory of her mother saying that she had no one. That memory was tied to powerful and intolerable feelings of loneliness and sadness, which had led Kathleen to engage in self-destructive behaviors as a way to manage her pain. She had never told her mother, and had held on to the memory and associated emotions for more than three years of suffering. When she was eventually ready to tell her mother, her mother broke down and cried, "You suffered for so long! Why didn't you ever tell me? Of course, I didn't mean that I was alone in relation to you. I'm so sad that you thought that." At fourteen Kathleen's amygdala and hippocampus had stored the memory of her mother's words, and that memory was attached to feeling hurt, sadness, and suffering.

The most consistent finding in imaging studies of people with BPD, compared to those without BPD, is increased activity in the amygdala, particularly if they also experience suicidal thoughts (Soloff et al. 2012). Finding a way to reduce this activity is critical to reducing the flow of unrelenting emotions in BPD.

Unregulated emotions are not always present. There are many situations in which your emotions are just fine. Context matters. This means that only certain people will experience your BPD. For instance you might be able to regulate your emotions at work so that they are not out of control when events are pretty neutral, yet you might not be able to regulate your emotions at home, when things get heated. This, too, can be confusing for others, who might argue that if you can do it in one place, then why not another? One way to explain it is to point out that the situation has changed. A person who is able to swim in a swimming pool is not able to do so if the water is boiling.

The Prefrontal Cortex

The prefrontal cortex (PFC) is the part of each brain hemisphere that is located right behind your forehead. It is responsible for controlling what are known as *executive functions*. Executive functions include the following:

- Mediating conflicting thoughts like *I want to eat more pizza because it tastes great; on the other hand I've already had three slices.*

- Making choices between right and wrong, or good and bad: *Should I call in sick to work, which means others will have to do more, but I can get a pedicure?*

- Predicting future events like *If I don't write the paper that's due tomorrow, I'll get a failing grade.*

- Governing social control, for example, suppressing the urge to pick your nose during dinner or to have sex with your significant other on the bus.

This brief brain-anatomy lesson is all you really need to know about the structures of the brain as they apply to BPD. Now we'll move on to how the amygdala and the PFC are supposed to work together.

Connecting the Amygdala and the PFC

Under typical circumstances, the PFC regulates the amygdala and the rest of the limbic system. So, for instance, imagine that you are wearing a light-colored jacket at a family reunion, and your hyperactive brother, who is excited to see you, trips and spills his glass of red wine all over you. Your amygdala processes the information, and you get angry at him. Your hippocampus kicks in as you remember all your years of having to deal with your brother's lack of body awareness, making you all the angrier. You want to lash out and yell at him. This is where your PFC steps in and says, *I know you want to yell at him, but it would ruin the reunion, and if you yell at him, he will get upset and not talk to you for a week. You can still be mad at him, but go get another jacket and talk to him later.*

These exchanges among the various parts of your brain happen very quickly, as fast as two hundred miles per hour; many of these communications happen without your awareness. Because your PFC is in charge of regulating your amygdala, you can see what would happen if your PFC were either not working well or not fully developed. You would have reduced ability to control the impulse to lash out. People with BPD are often called "impulsive," and as you will see later in this chapter, it's a fact that the PFC is not as developed in people with BPD as in those without BPD.

Brain Scans, Genes, and Neurotransmitters

The tests looking into the neurobiology of BPD that have received the most interest are brain scans, genetic mapping, and activity of *neurotransmitters*, which are also known as *brain chemicals*. We don't want to bury you under a mountain of studies, but we do think it's productive to show you where the research is pointing.

The Different Brain Scans

The following is an explanation of the different imaging and scanning techniques that are commonly used to study the brain.

- *Electroencephalogram* (EEG): This is a test that records the electrical activity of your brain. Electrodes are attached to your head and hooked by wires to a computer, which then records the activity. Different states of the brain show different electrical activity, so your sleeping brain looks very different from your brain when you are awake.

■ *Functional magnetic resonance imaging:* Also known as *functional MRI* (fMRI), this is a brain scan that uses powerful magnets to measure brain activity by detecting changes in blood flow. In other words, an fMRI could measure activity in your brain as you do things like talk or listen or think. This brain scan does not involve X-rays.

■ *Computerized tomography:* Often referred to as a *CAT scan,* this is an X-ray procedure that combines multiple X-ray images. With the aid of a computer, these X-ray images of your brain are then turned into three-dimensional images that show normal and abnormal structures.

■ *Positron emission tomography:* Also known as a *PET scan,* this is an imaging test that involves injecting a very small dose of a radioactive chemical into a vein in your arm. The chemical then travels to your brain and attaches to brain receptors. The radioactivity is then measured to give an indication of the level of activity in that part of the brain.

All of this research and these tests will make more sense when you see how mindfulness can influence biology.

What Brain Scans Show

Charles, a thirty-one-year-old grade-school teacher, came in looking for treatment because he had a hard time controlling his rage. He did well in the classroom, but with close friends and with dates, he would explode when he felt things weren't going his way or that people weren't being fair. He admitted that on a few occasions, he had yelled at his friends and, in desperate moments, physically attacked his girlfriends.

Charles is not unlike many of the people who come to see us because of impulsivity or aggression that's directed toward others or themselves. In research, behaviors such as self-mutilation, physical violence, assault, destruction of property, and drug use fall under the category of *impulsive aggression*, which is the one area in BPD that is well researched. In one study of violent offenders and impulsive fire setters, 47 percent were found to have a personality-disorder diagnosis, in particular, borderline and antisocial personality disorders (Virkkunen et al. 1996). In another study, male perpetrators of domestic violence were more likely to have a diagnosis of BPD than men who did not engage in domestic violence (Dutton, Starzomski, and Ryan 1996).

Brain Scans and Aggression

Brain scans show that people with impulsive aggression have lower levels of activity in the PFC (Spoont 1992). People with BPD also have less brain activity in the PFC (Goyer et al. 1994). What both of these studies show is that the PFC is not as active in people who display impulsive aggression. Most brain-scanning studies reveal that people with BPD show disordered functioning in the PFC, compared to people without BPD, and this is particularly true if the person with BPD also suffers from PTSD. As we noted earlier, having a less-active PFC means having a more difficult time with regulating emotions (like anger).

Genes

One of the largest studies on BPD and genetics looked at 92 identical and 129 nonidentical Norwegian twin pairs. The researchers found that genes accounted for 69 percent of the symptoms of BPD and that environmental factors accounted for the other 31 percent (Torgersen 2000). Most researchers consider BPD to be roughly 60 percent genetic and 40 percent environmental. This might lead you to think that because of your genes, you are destined to have BPD, but mindfulness can change how you respond to things. In any case mindfulness can certainly help with the 40 percent of BPD symptoms that your environment contributes to.

Another finding in genetic studies of BPD is that you can inherit impulsive aggression (Coccaro, Bergeman, and McClearn 1993).

Neurotransmitters

In this section we will discuss three brain chemicals that have been studied in BPD so that you can understand why they are important to know about and, later, how mindfulness might help to regulate them.

Opiates

Under ordinary circumstances, in response to any body-tissue damage, the brain releases *opiates* to dull the pain. These opiates that the brain creates are similar to opiate painkillers that are available by prescription. It appears that people with BPD who self-injure have lower levels of natural opiates compared to people with BPD who don't self-injure (Stanley et al. 2010). Many people who take opiate painkillers report a feeling of wellness, so one theory is that the reason some people with BPD self-injure is to increase their levels of natural opiates in order to feel better. And in fact many people with BPD who self-injure state that they do feel better, even if just briefly, after engaging in the behavior (Simeon et al. 1992).

Research shows that if you have BPD and self-injure, you won't perceive pain as much as someone without BPD does (Bohus et al. 2000). This means that the self-injury (like cutting) that would typically cause someone without BPD to feel pain might not cause you as much pain. However, people with BPD have more pain syndromes, such as headaches and muscle, abdominal, and back pain, than those without BPD (Tragesser, Bruns, and Disorbio 2010).

How do we explain the apparent contradiction that when people with BPD cut, they feel less pain, yet they have more pain syndromes? The issue is that most self-injury occurs in the context of high emotional distress, and during those moments, perception of physical pain is diminished. When you are not emotionally dysregulated, you can experience the pain that others experience—or even more, based on the research that shows that people with BPD have more pain syndromes than other people do. One of the reasons people with BPD have more pain syndromes is that overall, people with BPD tend to be in poorer health than those without BPD (Frankenburg and Zanarini 2004).

Serotonin

Serotonin is a brain chemical that plays an important role in the regulation of mood, sleep, and learning. It is found throughout the brain and the digestive system, and has been implicated in depression, suicide, anxiety, and appetite regulation. Some people with depression and anxiety actually feel their symptoms in their stomachs, and if you are too anxious, you might be susceptible to irritable bowel syndrome (Dorn et al. 2007), likely because of serotonin. Many studies show that people with BPD have low levels of serotonin activity and that this is associated with impulsive aggression (Goodman and New 2000). Research also shows that low serotonin activity is associated with suicide attempts (Lidberg et al. 2000) and self-injury (New et al. 1997).

You might have heard of medications that increase the amount of serotonin in your brain. These medications can be very helpful in reducing depression and anxiety, but they are not totally without side effects. Sometimes if you increase the amount of serotonin too much, you can feel *more* suicidal.

Cortisol

Cortisol is a chemical released during stress that helps to break down carbohydrates and proteins in order to increase the supply of glucose and oxygen in your muscles, the heart, and the brain. However, when you have a lot of stress over a long period of time, a high level of cortisol leads to an increase in blood pressure and an increase in sugar levels, which in turn leads to unhealthy fat building up in your abdomen. It also leads to thinning of your bones and prevents collagen from forming. *Collagen* is the molecule that makes connective tissue, and it is essential for healing any skin damage. Another downside of high cortisol levels is that it suppresses immune-system response and causes your body to age faster. Also, long-term exposure to high levels of cortisol damages and reduces the number of cells in your hippocampus, which is, as you will recall, your brain's primary memory center.

As if all of the negative effects of high levels of cortisol from stress weren't enough, research shows not only that people with BPD have high levels of cortisol (Wingenfeld et al. 2007), but also that these high levels predict a higher risk of suicide over time (Lester and Bean 1992).

The Neurobiology of Mindfulness

Now that you have some understanding of how your brain, your genes, and your brain chemicals might interact in ways that lead to BPD, we will examine the biology of mindfulness and tie it to the biology of BPD. If mindfulness is going to help you out of your suffering, then it has to influence the regions and chemicals of the brain that we just looked at.

Strengthen Your PFC

Mindfulness practice that focuses on paying attention activates the prefrontal cortex, the part of the brain that doesn't seem to work all that well in BPD (Brefczynski-Lewis et al. 2007; Newberg et al. 2001; Newberg and Iversen 2003). It turns out that different types of mindfulness activate the PFC in different ways. This is similar to different physical exercises changing your body in different ways. However, just as almost any exercise is healthy for your body, the different types of mindfulness all help to keep your brain focused, attentive, and aware. All of these practices will strengthen the attentional circuits in your PFC and reduce the reactivity of your amygdala, meaning that you can choose the mindfulness practice that works for you and your lifestyle.

Meditation and Yoga

Mindfulness meditation is a practice that generally is taught initially with a focus on breathing. As the practice develops, the practitioner moves from focused attention to a broadening of awareness. The focus on the breath is a core practice in many forms of mindfulness, including that which is practiced in DBT. This form of meditation has been shown to strengthen brain activity in the prefrontal cortex, particularly in the attention areas and the parts of the prefrontal cortex that are involved in impulse control (Hölzel et al. 2007).

Transcendental Meditation (TM) is a twenty-minute practice that is usually done twice daily. You obtain a specific, personal mantra through The Transcendental Meditation Program. During the meditation, your eyes are closed and you focus your attention on the mantra you have been given.

People who practice certain forms of meditation and yoga can experience a calming effect all over the body while meditating. EEG studies indicate that as meditators sit quietly, their brain activity begins to slow. For TM this slowing occurs in the frontal lobes and near the midline of the brain (Wallace, Benson, and Wilson 1971). Certain forms of yoga showed similar brain results (Corby et al. 1978; Elson, Hauri, and Cunis 1977). During TM and certain forms of yoga, your brain will slow down, which leads to lower anxiety and has a calming effect. Yoga has also been shown to increase activity in the prefrontal cortex and decrease activity in the amygdala, both of which are of particular interest in BPD (Cohen et al. 2009).

As we saw in chapter 2, various religions use forms of *meditative prayer*. Christian contemplative prayer has been the focus of two imaging studies. In the first study, six religion teachers from a Christian community underwent a PET scan while entering a mindfulness state by reciting Psalm 23 from the Bible. Their scans were compared to six nonreligious volunteers. The teachers showed higher activity in the parts of the frontal lobe associated with attention than did the volunteers (Azari et al. 2001). In the second study (Newberg and Iversen 2003), scans were obtained from three nuns who had practiced *centering prayer* for fifteen years. In centering prayer the focus is on a prayer or phrase from the Bible, which is meant to help the person achieve the experience of being in the presence of God. Compared to when the nuns were not praying, during mindful prayer their brains showed higher amounts of blood flow to various regions of the frontal lobe.

Zazen is also known as the "sitting meditation" of Zen Buddhism. We have both done five-day zazen retreats where we don't speak for the entire time and sit for up to sixteen hours a day. We encourage you to start with just ten to twenty minutes a day. During the practice of zazen, you sit cross-legged on a round cushion, with your hands on your lap. You keep your eyes open, casting your gaze toward the floor a few feet in front of you. Traditionally you would focus on a Buddhist teaching; however, in a secular practice it's typical to focus on the rise and fall of your breath. Three EEG studies of meditators practicing zazen showed a marked calming of the brain (Kubota et al. 2001; Murata et al. 2004; Takahashi et al. 2005).

How Mindfulness Changes the BPD Brain

Although mindfulness is a component of various psychotherapies these days—therapies like DBT, Mindfulness-Based Stress Reduction (MBSR), and mindfulness-based cognitive therapy (MBCT)—there is very little research on its use as a stand-alone skill to treat BPD. In fact only one study has looked at mindfulness in BPD (Sauer and Baer 2011).

In the study the forty participants with BPD were instructed to write for ten minutes about a situation that had made them very angry. The researchers looked at the short-term effects of mindful, self-focused attention on the ability of people with BPD to tolerate the distress of ruminative thoughts such as *Why do people treat me this way?* Each participant was then randomly assigned to engage in the ruminative thoughts or in mindful self-focus for several minutes, and then they were given a distress-tolerance task. The mindfulness group persisted significantly longer than the rumination group on the distress-tolerance task and reported significantly lower levels of anger after the self-focus period.

Mindfulness and Other Common Problems

Even though there is only one study on the dedicated use of mindfulness in BPD, there are many studies on the use of mindfulness for symptoms commonly experienced by people who have BPD.

Pain, Physical Illness, and Neurotransmitters

People who struggle with BPD have higher levels of physical illness and experience more pain syndromes than the general population. As a consequence they take more pain medication than average (Frankenburg and Zanarini 2004). Mindfulness has been shown (Zeidan et al. 2011) to:

- change the unpleasant physical sensation of the pain itself;

- change emotional reactions to the pain, such as fear and anger;

- change the thoughts that are triggered by the pain. Typical thoughts are *This pain will never end* and *I'm going to suffer for the rest of my life.*

The way in which mindfulness meditation is thought to change the pain experience is, in part, that when the PFC is activated, one of the chemicals it produces is β-endorphin, a painkilling opiate. This leads to not only a reduction in the sense of pain, but also a reduction in breathing rate, a decrease in the sense of fear, and an increase in the experience of joy (Newberg and Iversen 2003).

If you have difficulty paying attention, high levels of stress, and a compromised immune system, mindfulness helps those too (Tang et al. 2007). For instance, earlier in the chapter, we saw how excess cortisol can take a toll on the body. Many studies have reported that mindful meditation leads to a reduction in cortisol levels (Carlson et al. 2004; Sudsuang, Chentanez, and Veluvan 1991).

Anxiety, Depression, OCD, Substance Abuse, and More

Many people with BPD have what are known as co-occurring, or *comorbid*, conditions, so it would not be unusual for your psychiatrist or psychologist to say that besides BPD, you have a mood disorder, an anxiety disorder, a substance-use disorder, or some other condition. Fortunately there are many studies that show that mindfulness helps for many of these conditions; for instance, mindfulness-based therapies help in the treatment of anxiety (Kabat-Zinn et al. 1992; Miller, Fletcher, and Kabat-Zinn 1995), obsessive-compulsive disorder (Schwartz and Begley 2002), and depression (Teasdale et al. 2000; Ma and Teasdale 2004).

Also, as you read earlier, serotonin is the chemical of happiness, and typically psychiatrists prescribe medications that increase serotonin when you are depressed. There is no evidence that these medications work for BPD, even though serotonin appears to be low in people with BPD. Low levels of serotonin are highly associated with suicide (Li and He 2007). If medications aren't helping, then it's critical to find other ways to increase serotonin in the brain, and researchers are doing just that. To date there are no studies that show that mindfulness leads to an increase in serotonin; however, there is research that shows that the stories we recall can increase seratonin levels. In one study participants were asked to recall sad, happy, and neutral stories from their pasts, with the goal of inducing sadness, happiness, and neutral emotions. Their brains were then scanned for serotonin activity and showed that serotonin went up when they told stories that induced happiness and went down during stories that induced sadness (Perreau-Linck et al. 2007). Thus, being mindful of stories that bring you joy could, in fact, boost your seratonin.

Meditation, Not Medication

Never been mindful? Even if you are totally new to mindfulness, you will experience positive effects. One study of 174 people who had never practiced mindfulness found almost immediate benefits in the form of reduced stress, decreased medical symptoms, and increased overall well-being after just eight weeks of mindfulness practice, consisting of one session per week, lasting two and one-half hours each (Carmody and Baer 2008).

In this chapter we have seen that both BPD and mindfulness are functions of the brain. In order to treat BPD, you might consider taking medication; however, this approach has its drawbacks. There is a limit to the amount of medication you can take and when you can take it, and many medications come with significant side effects. On the other hand, you can practice mindfulness at any time of day or night, it has no side effects, it helps for many different conditions, and it costs you no money, unless you are paying for mindfulness training.

Mindfulness is a skill that you can develop, and we will show you how in the next part of the book. According to a national survey (Barnes, Bloom, and Nahin 2008), mindfulness practice increased from 7.6 percent in 2002 to 9.4 percent in 2007, making it one of the most commonly used "alternative" therapies. This means that nearly thirty million American meditators are recognizing the benefit of the practice. If you have BPD, you, too, will find that mindfulness is a transformative practice. It is associated with functional and structural brain changes that lead to positive emotions, a reduction in pain, and improved overall health, which is not something that can be said for many therapies. We will now move on to part 2, where we will teach you how to practice mindfulness.

Part 2

The How and What
of Mindfulness

Chapter 4

The Practice of Mindfulness

Imagine trying to learn something new without being given any instructions when learning what to do or how to do it. For most of us, many things would be nearly impossible to do. When learning to drive a car, play tennis, or knit, it's much easier to have someone coach you through the necessary steps of what to do and how to do it. Mindfulness is the core skill of DBT, and the next two chapters teach you how to practice this skill. Part 3 will help you learn, step-by step, how to use your mindfulness skills to address specific symptoms of BPD.

Perhaps you, like many people suffering from BPD, are skeptical of the idea that mindfulness can help. We asked a twenty-three-year-old mother of two young children who has struggled with BPD for as long as she can remember what her initial thoughts were when we suggested that she practice mindfulness, and this was her response:

> *I thought,* How can something so (seemingly) simple bring relief to such unrelenting misery and suffering? What the hell is mindfulness? This doctor is on crack. Next doctor, please. *When you think of mindfulness, you think of meditation and Zen and Buddhist principles, and kind of immediately dismiss it as being weird and reserved for dorks or monks. Especially when you're at the lowest point of your life (which you have to admit is where a lot of people are when they come to therapy), it's almost impossible to believe that this weird idea is a necessary part of recovery.*

It makes sense to have these types of reservations about the idea of practicing mindfulness. How can something like paying attention to your breath relieve suffering? Much of the confusion and misunderstanding come from simply not knowing what the practice of mindfulness is or how to do it.

Knowing what to do makes it easier, but simply knowing what to do without practicing is nearly useless. Knowing that you have to hold the steering wheel and step on the accelerator doesn't mean that you know how to drive a car. You have to practice, and practice takes time. One way to think about it is as exercising the "mindfulness muscle" in your brain. Many people with BPD find themselves using short-term solutions (cutting themselves, driving recklessly, and engaging in disordered eating and other potentially destructive behaviors) to solve long-term problems. These solutions can provide quick, though temporary, relief from suffering, but generally cause more problems and ultimately a return to suffering. The practice of mindfulness provides a long-term solution to suffering, but the journey takes time and patience.

Setting Up Your Mindfulness Practice

You may be wondering how long and how often you should practice mindfulness. For the purposes of this book and for people who are just starting out, we recommend practicing a minimum of twenty minutes each day, which can be divided into two ten-minute sessions. Once you have been practicing for a while, try to increase the duration of your practice gradually, working up to thirty minutes or more each day. Keep in mind that we will be teaching you ways to use mindfulness throughout your day, but carving out time for a formal meditation practice is key to learning this skill and integrating it into your life. No matter how skilled at mindfulness you become, you must remain committed to practicing for a prescribed period each day.

When is a good time to practice? This is a matter of preference. Some people like to begin the day with mindfulness practice, while others prefer practicing in the afternoon or before going to bed. The most important thing is to make a commitment and stick to it. If you know that you are someone who puts things off or returns home in the evening quite tired, you will likely be more successful with practicing first thing in the morning. The goal is to develop a habit of practicing mindfulness, so committing to a specific time will help you do this. You may find it useful to set an alert on your cell phone or computer, or leave yourself a note.

Some people find it important to practice in the same location every day. We will be teaching you a number of different types of practice with the goal of enabling you to practice anywhere. Think about what was helpful for you in the past when you created a new routine in your life.

People who are starting mindfulness practice also wonder how or if they are supposed to sit. We will teach you many different types of practices, some in which you will be seated and others in which you will move around. Sitting in a formal lotus position is definitely not required.

For sitting practices, find a seated position in which your chest remains open (without crossing your arms) and your sit bones make even contact with the surface you're sitting on. Specifically, sit up straight in a chair—using pillows behind your back if needed—with both of your feet firmly on the floor and without crossing your legs or ankles. Or sit cross-legged on the floor. Draw your shoulders back and rest your arms gently on your lap, palms up if that's comfortable. Don't cross your arms or hunch over. Part of the practice is to pay attention to how you are sitting. Finally, you will do most of the mindfulness practices with your eyes open; we live most of our lives with open eyes, so your practice should be as you live.

Taking Control of Your Mind

The practice of mindfulness allows you to take control of your mind. You may feel tossed around or consumed by your feelings, and imagine that there's nothing you can do about it. In DBT this is sometimes referred to as *emotion mind*, where our emotions dictate our actions

(Linehan 1993). Like others with BPD, you may find that you are dragged around by powerful feelings and that sometimes the consequences can be grim. What's worse is that when you look back on these times, you can't always figure out how you got there. When you don't pay attention, your feelings can make you change your mind and not stick to your commitments. You might end important relationships and even do or say things that go against your own values.

> Lisa, a bright, articulate, and kind twenty-year-old with BPD with whom we have worked on mindfulness for the last two and a half years, frequently found herself thrown about by her feelings and engaging in "mood-dependent behaviors"; that is, her goals, commitments, and relationships would change rapidly depending on her mood. This was an exhausting way to live. Lisa would find herself sending e-mails to her mother, brother, and boyfriend, detailing her intense hatred of them. Sometimes this happened after arguments or feelings of disappointment, and other times the e-mails seemingly came out of nowhere. She complained that people said she was "too much to handle." Her decisions and conclusions were driven by her emotions, and rational thinking appeared to go out the window.
>
> The problem was that within hours, her emotions changed such that she was riddled with guilt and shame over her behavior and the intense fear that she had caused irreparable damage to a relationship. This type of suffering reinforced her feelings that she was a terrible person who caused others pain. Lisa felt that this was a horrible way to live, and we agreed. How did a relationship that was so important one moment suddenly become unnecessary and intolerable the next? Getting tossed around by your emotions can be incredibly painful and destructive.

Most of us don't pay attention to the habitual nature of our thinking. We don't pay attention, because we have not been taught how to do so, which was how it was for Lisa before she began learning mindfulness. An untrained mind can cause significant distress, even without your knowing it. You may find that your thinking falls into one of two extremes. On one end, you get so tangled up in your thoughts that you pay too much attention to specific thoughts or worries to the point where you cannot think about much else or see the bigger picture. At the other end, you pay very little attention at all to how you think. Perhaps you tend to feel as if things "just happened," and cannot figure out how events unfolded or what led up to your reaction. Each of these extremes can lead to problems. When you are unable to figure out how feelings, thoughts, and events unfold, you get stuck in suffering. Awareness, attention, and curiosity allow you to take control of your thinking and your responses so that you can break these patterns.

Why should you pay attention and be curious? A lack of attention and curiosity keeps all of us living routine and habitual lives, and can create distance from painful thoughts and feelings. This may seem like a good thing or may even be your goal at times, but it's not an effective long-term solution. Keeping your distance from your emotions may be driving your suffering. Paying attention to thinking means slowing down and looking in detail at your thoughts: the speed of your thoughts (*Are my thought racing or sluggish?*), quality of your thoughts (*Are my thoughts organized or jumping around from one subject to another like a monkey leaping from tree to tree?*), tone of your thoughts (*Are my thoughts angry, judgmental, kind?*), and the actual content of your thoughts. (*What I am thinking about? Dinner, my partner, the fight with my boss*).

As a goal of this practice, people who develop mindfulness learn to take control of their thoughts and feelings. By paying attention, you can find more joy, peace, and serenity in the way you live. Learning how to do this can free you from the chaos and stress in your mind. For someone who has never practiced mindfulness, freedom from chaos can be pretty hard to imagine.

Practicing Mindfulness

Through mindfulness practice, you will learn how to attend to what's going on in your mind and body, and once you do that, you can learn different things to do with your thoughts and feelings that will decrease your suffering. In DBT, these activities are called the "what" and "how" skills (Linehan 1993), that is, what you do to be mindful and how you do it.

Throughout this chapter we will give you specific practices that will focus on each aspect of mindfulness. We would like for you to try each practice at least once and keep a journal to record your experience as your practice. You may find that you enjoy some practices more than others, but it's important to expose yourself to as many types of mindfulness practice as possible because you never know what might be helpful if don't try. Remember, it's not necessarily about liking the practice, but about challenging your mind and being curious. It's also important to remember that on some days, you may feel more successful than on other days. We are always amazed at how we can practice one day and attend to it with little effort, while on other days, the same practice feels impossible. With mindfulness, your experience is always changing. Remember, your mind will wander often; when you notice that your mind has wandered, bring your attention back to the task of just being mindful. The act of returning your mind to the task is exercising your mindfulness muscle.

Use Intention

The practice of mindfulness in any moment begins with intention. Anything that you can do mindlessly, you can do mindfully, but what makes the practice mindful is your intention to do it mindfully. Practice doesn't "just happen." You get to choose. You can get in your car and drive to work on autopilot, thinking about your upcoming day, how desperate you are for another cup of coffee, or whether you will have time to go to the gym after work. Or instead you can decide that your intention when you drive will be just to drive. You will notice your desire for coffee, and refocus on driving. If you choose to practice your mindfulness skills, it is with the intention to practice. As you drive, notice your mind wandering, and if it does, bring it back to driving. It's amazing what you can notice when you turn such a habitual daily task into a mindfulness practice. It is mindfulness if you are aware that you are practicing.

Some people who begin practicing mindfulness tell us that they have heard that the goal of mindfulness is to have their minds never wander. It's impossible for your mind not to wander. As we mentioned earlier, our brains produce thoughts. It's one of the things the brain is designed to do. The act of mindfulness is choosing, with intention, to return your mind to the task you set out to do. Each time your mind wanders and you intentionally bring it back, you are being mindful. Mindfulness is not simply about having a quiet mind.

Decide to Practice

When you decide to practice mindfulness, remind yourself that you are beginning a mindfulness practice. When you are new to mindfulness, it's important to explicitly tell yourself that you are about to do something mindfully—for example, *I'm going to mindfully wash the dishes for the next five to ten minutes*. This provides a cue to your brain that you are embarking on a practice and choosing where to focus your mind.

Do Something Different Each Day

Practice the skill of intention by setting an intention to change one of your habitual behaviors each day for one week. For example, for an entire day, intentionally cross your legs with your nondominant leg on top, brush your teeth with your nondominant hand, change the order in which you carry out your morning or bedtime routine, take a different route to work or school, or carry your purse or briefcase in your nondominant hand. The idea is to practice intentionally doing something differently, committing to do so for a specific period, and then paying attention to what you observe.

Watch and Notice

The second mindfulness skill that you will learn is to simply watch and notice your thoughts and feelings. This is known as the "observe" skill in DBT (Linehan 1993). In the context of mindfulness, to watch means to just notice without putting labels on the experience. It is noting and attending to the experience with all of your senses. Because we typically label experiences, mastery of this skill can be challenging.

All too often, we do things without really paying attention, so we miss critical information. Earlier we mentioned that watching and noticing means paying attention. When you pay attention, you will begin to recognize the automatic responses that you have to most situations, and for people with BPD, it is often these automatic, habitual responses in relationships that cause so much misery. We once had a client who got angry every time his mother spoke. He would get angry whether she said "Good morning" to him or "nagged" him about cleaning up his room. He said that it was just her voice that made him angry. He had become so annoyed with her that he automatically responded negatively, whether she was doing or saying something that bothered him, or doing or saying something kind. Paying attention to these automatic responses allowed him to take control of how he responded to her, and ultimately taught him that he had a choice in how he responded to any situation in his life.

Learning to observe the early signs of emotions in your body can help you to not be so surprised or overwhelmed by an intense emotion that it feels as if it came out of nowhere.

The act of simply watching or observing can quiet the mind. Don't underestimate how challenging it is to not use words. In our culture we tend to put words to all of our experiences. Imagine sitting in your room and just observing the sounds in your house, just noticing the sounds without labeling what they are. Or imagine sitting outside, watching the sunset without getting caught up in the exact colors, just watching as they become less and less vibrant. Or imagine watching clouds in the sky as they move past and change shapes. The act of watching and noticing turns off the thinking part of your mind, which gets revved up in times of stress and anxiety. Watching and noticing can be an excellent way to calm your mind and body. You can think of it as letting your mind be in a state of "being" instead of a state of thinking and doing. Let your mind just be with what you notice.

Once you get the hang of attending by watching and noticing things outside of you, you will increasingly be able to watch your own thoughts without getting caught up in the content or action urges that arise. Our minds get busier and our worries stronger when we get caught up in these thoughts. Just watching thoughts go by like cans on a conveyer belt can actually slow down the mind. This means that you need to let go of problem solving and understanding, and simply watch. It's as if you were standing on a platform in a train station and watching trains come in and out of the station, but never getting on.

One day Elizabeth, who had been in treatment for BPD with us and working on mindfulness for about a year, said:

> *I get what you've been talking about! You won't believe how many thoughts and feelings I had in five minutes when I was waiting for a friend, and I didn't even get out of the chair! If I had acted on my thoughts, I would have made my situation pretty bad and done what I always do when I find myself thinking this way. First, I noticed excitement that we were having lunch together. Then I heard her talking to someone in the front of the restaurant, and felt devastated that she liked that girl's company better. Then I felt empty and angry. Finally I concluded that I was not important and she didn't care about me; otherwise she would have come directly to the table. This quickly led me to think, I'm not worth caring for and don't deserve love from others. I felt pretty bad. Then I had the intense urge to leave the restaurant and walk right by her without saying a word, because I was sure that if she cared about me, she would run after me.*
>
> *I noticed this urge but realized that these were all just thoughts and feelings for which I had little evidence. These thoughts continued for a bit, and within a few moments, she came to the table, was happy to see me, and apologized that she had gotten "stuck" talking to a family friend who happened to be at*

*the restaurant. And again, my mood shifted. I realized that had
I left, she would have been totally confused and not gone after me,
and I would have felt miserable.*

Just as your stomach produces digestive enzymes, your brain produces thoughts. That's what brains do, and there's nothing wrong with thoughts. You don't judge your stomach for producing enzymes, but you probably often judge your thoughts. You can attend to thoughts without taking any action at all. You don't need to listen to all of your thoughts or, for that matter, believe them. With practice, watching your thoughts go by can slow them down. You may find great pleasure in being able to turn down the running commentary of a busy mind or no longer needing to constantly react to your thoughts.

What Makes Our Minds So Busy

There are times when having a very busy mind can be distracting and unpleasant. Take rumination for instance. *Rumination*, in psychology, is the process of spending a lot of time thinking about a situation. For some, rumination can be difficult to control. You can spend hours and hours thinking about a situation over and over again, which can lead to obsession, depression, and fear. Some of our clients with BPD are perfectionists, so, for example, they might spend so much time thinking about how to perfect a term paper that they never even write down a single word.

Another type of busy mind is catastrophizing. As you will recall from chapter 1, catastrophizing is a type of thinking that leads you to believe that something is far worse than it actually is and that all of the possible outcomes will lead to disaster. So, taking the example of the term paper, catastrophizing thoughts would go like this: *I can't write the paper, so I'll fail the course and won't get a recommendation. I won't be accepted to college, so I can't go to graduate school. Therefore I won't get a good job and will be a failure for the rest of my life!*

One young man began with the thought that he would do poorly at a job interview, and that thought led him to the conclusion that he would end up homeless and living under a bridge. We can laugh as we look back on it now, but the amount of stress and anxiety that this type of thinking causes cannot be overstated.

One of the joys of mindfulness is that you can develop the capacity to get some distance from your thoughts, and maybe even laugh at where your mind goes. One benefit of mindfulness is learning to not take yourself so seriously.

Using Your Senses

You can watch and notice with all of your senses. Note that everything you watch or attend to changes, whether it's pleasant or not, and you can watch that happen. The practice of using your senses is probably the easiest way to understand this. Get a scented flower and smell its fragrance. Put a sour candy in your mouth and hold it there for a while, experience the taste, and observe how it changes. Sit outside wearing short sleeves and notice the temperature on your skin. Sit on a park bench and, without turning your head or shifting your gaze, simply watch as people walk in and out of your line of sight. Don't follow them with your eyes; just observe them coming in and out of view. Holding your attention, noticing when you get distracted, and bringing yourself back to these experiences is mindfulness.

Do Nothing but Watch and Attend

Many of us are tempted to do something, rather than simply observe what's happening. How often do you not scratch an itch? The desire to do something comes very strongly, especially when your thoughts come with strong emotions. Thoughts and feelings are often followed by an urge to do something. In DBT we focus quite a bit on action urges, because an important function of emotion is to motivate or prompt actions and behaviors. The behavior is not part of the emotion, but the urge is (Linehan 1993).

Sometimes we have urges that prompt behaviors that are not useful, that get in the way of our goals, or that have negative consequences. It's important to be able to identify the emotion and the urge and not always act on it. To develop this capacity, we are asking you to intentionally notice the urge and do nothing about it. We have urges all of the time. How often do you find yourself at a store becoming angry or impatient at the salesperson for being unable to help you? The urge may be to yell at the person or treat him badly. However, if you need to purchase an item and this is the only salesclerk who can help you, yelling can create a lot of suffering for you and result in the salesperson not helping you. In an extreme case you could end up being escorted out of the store, unable to purchase the item you came in for.

Can you remember any times when not reacting to an urge would have been more effective, but you just couldn't figure out how to avoid reacting? This is where just watching and attending can help.

Typical human reactions to thoughts and emotions tend to fall into one of two opposing categories: suppression and enhancement.

Suppression. If you have a thought or urge, one reaction would be to suppress that thought. This is like squashing down a thought by thinking things like *I shouldn't have that thought. That's a bad thought to have; what an awful thought.* The problem with this approach is that it often increases the intensity of the thought or urge, making it even more powerful. It would be like our telling you, "Don't think about a pink balloon, and don't think about a pink balloon right now!" While you may have no interest in pink balloons at all, once we tell you to not think about pink balloons, suddenly pink balloons will be in your mind all of the time. (Are you still thinking of pink balloons?)

Enhancement. Enhancement is the opposite of suppression, when instead of pushing away a painful thought or urge, you end up magnifying it, which also leads to suffering. In this case, you find yourself acting on urges that increase the intensity of your thoughts and feelings, and doing so without awareness.

Pitfalls to Reacting rather than Watching and Noticing

A common pitfall to reacting to your thoughts and emotions rather than noticing them is that you tend to "collect evidence"—in the form of thoughts, memories, experiences, or cognitive distortions—that validates how you are feeling in the present moment. Collecting evidence, one-sided as it may be, that you are loathsome or miserable will simply lead to more suffering.

> Lisa, who was introduced earlier, frequently found herself enhancing the exact emotions that she found the most distressing, and discovered that she had been doing so for years without any awareness. She was unable to just watch and notice these thoughts without acting on them. An avid journal writer, in times of distress Lisa would find herself spending hours rereading her journal to "make sure I remember that I'm messed up and ruin people's lives." She would spend hours reading and thinking about everything that would validate her current emotional state. This behavior resulted in missed college classes, missed outings with friends, inability to get out of bed, hopelessness, and thoughts of suicide. Her behavior was enticing, because it validated her suffering, even though she didn't particularly like what she was doing.

Mindfully paying attention allows you to be in control of your mind, rather than the other way around. This skill of watching and noticing will teach you about who you are and how your mind works. It is the key to knowing yourself and all of your thoughts and feelings.

As you start to practice mindfulness, you will become more aware of not only unpleasant and painful emotions, but also wonderful and pleasant experiences that you previously missed. One man with BPD who had started a mindfulness practice came in after a few weeks beaming, declaring that this was the first time in seventeen years that he had ever noticed the beauty of the Charles River, even though he had lived next to it all his life. Just noticing the river brought him a joy that he had not previously experienced. Even those of us who practice mindfulness daily have opportunities to observe things that we previously missed. Gillian has been getting coffee at the hospital cafeteria every day for the last three years. Recently she looked up and noticed a huge, colorful mural on the wall that she had never seen before. She noted, "When I think back on it, most days I rush into the cafeteria, thinking about all that I have to do during the day, and routinely get my coffee without ever shifting my gaze to look at what's around me." When we get lost in our thoughts, we often miss what's right in front of us.

People often express excitement as they begin to notice pleasant experiences, but wonder if it's worth it to experience the pain of paying attention to hurtful emotions and experiences. You might argue that awareness of the experience of suffering is exactly the reason why you don't want to practice mindfulness. If you are like many others, noticing painful emotional experiences will motivate you to stop noticing or to take action to change the experience. This is completely natural, yet the practice will lead you to see that all thoughts and feelings change, whether you like them or not, and usually when you pay attention to them, they can change more quickly if you would like them to.

It's All in Your Head

An interesting fact of brain neurology is that emotions that are left alone (not suppressed or enhanced) last for a very short time, somewhere between five and twenty seconds. If you could train your mind to simply observe, five to twenty seconds would be all you would need to endure an unpleasant emotion. When you think about the painful situation over and over again, you could stretch those thoughts from twenty seconds to minutes, hours, days, and even months and years. Learning to let things go would allow you to suffer less. Buddhist meditators have known this for more than two thousand years, and central to their belief is that the origin of suffering is attachment, or holding on. For many of us, rather than letting thoughts and emotions pass, we hold on, react, and suffer. Learning to attend to your mind by watching and noticing is the first step in learning to let go.

Let Thoughts and Feelings Go by Just Watching Them

If you simply watch and attend, you will notice that experiences, feelings, and thoughts arise in your mind and then slip out away like clouds moving across the sky. The thoughts and feelings may return, like clouds when the wind changes direction. Your goal is to let the thoughts and feelings go, rather than cling to them. When we cling to our thoughts and feelings, they stay with us. When thoughts stick in your mind, it's usually because they have powerful emotions attached to them. Imagine thinking of an orange. Usually the thought of an orange wouldn't stick around in your mind for a long time, but if, when you were a child, other kids had thrown oranges at you during every recess, the thought of an orange might be a painful one that might stick in your head for a while. Many people have had painful experiences that stick in their minds, and this is because of the emotions associated with these experiences. It makes perfect sense that memories can be very hard to let go of. Learning to let them go is a hard thing to do and yet ultimately essential if suffering is to be reduced. It's also important to remember that you can always go back to your thoughts and memories. The goal is to be able to choose when you want to think about something and when you don't.

Watching and noticing is a way to expose yourself to the emotions that you find difficult to bear so that you can get better at bearing them. Charlotte was terrified of using public transportation. Slowly, we exposed her to thoughts and images of buses and trains, and got her to attend to her thoughts by watching and noticing the fear that arose. We also had her sit with the fear without distracting herself from it or doing something to end it. Eventually she was able to get on a bus, which allowed her to become more independent.

In mindfulness practice, watching and attending means attending to exactly what is. This means attending to everything that's happening in this very moment, leaving nothing out and adding nothing to it. Thoughts, feelings, and sensations will come and go. Everything changes. In every moment, notice what is, and you also will notice that things change.

Watching and attending to an experience is different from the experience itself. You can liken this to watching a movie or going to a baseball game. *Watching* a movie is different from being *in* the movie. Watching a baseball game is different from playing in the game. You are not your thoughts. You are not your feelings. You are not your desires or emotions, and you can watch all of them come and go.

Mindfulness Practice: Taste

Place a raisin, a mint, or a piece of chocolate in your mouth and hold it there for two minutes. Notice the texture and taste during the experience. Bring your attention to this activity and watch how your experience changes over time. Notice the thoughts and feelings that come into your mind. When your mind wanders to other thoughts, return your attention to what you have in your mouth.

■

Mindfulness Practice: Smell

Take a flower or fragrant cream, and notice its scent for two minutes. Move the item closer to and farther away from you. Does the scent change? Remember, when your mind wanders, notice this and bring your attention back to watching the item and smelling the scent. Pay attention to specific thoughts that arise in your mind throughout the experience.

■

Mindfulness Practice: Touch

There are a number of ways to practice mindfulness using touch. Place your hands together, lining up your fingers and palms so that they are pressing together. Now slide your hands back and forth against one another for twenty seconds. Notice the sensation and the temperature as you rub. Stop rubbing your hands together, and for thirty seconds more, notice the sensation in your hands. A second practice is to spend two minutes noticing an itch without scratching it. Pay attention to the changing sensations in each of these practices. Do each of these practices for two to three minutes.

■

Mindfulness Practice: Sound

Sit outside in a park or in your front yard or backyard for twenty minutes. See if you can pick up the sounds of nature about you. Just notice them as sounds, without spending time trying to figure out what they are. Is the sound loud or soft, high or low pitched?

■

Mindfulness Practice: Sight

Spend two to three minutes examining your hand as if you've never seen it before. The idea with this practice is to examine and attend to your hand and all that you see. Look at the front and back of your hand. Notice your fingers and the lines and shades of your skin. Our hands are so integral to our day-to-day lives, and we pay very little attention to them. The saying goes, "I know it like the back of my hand," but how many of us actually know the backs of our hands?

■

Label

We have introduced the skill of watching and noticing, and now we will move on to the next skill: "labeling," putting words to your experience. Labeling allows us to categorize our experiences and communicate them with others and ourselves. Similarly, DBT uses the "describe" skill as a way of putting words to your experience (Linehan 1993). The skills of noticing (which you can practice by itself) and labeling are often used together; you must first be able to notice your thoughts and feelings, and then you can learn to mindfully label them. Many find this mindfulness practice a bit easier to grasp than merely noticing. Labeling is a very important skill, because it is often the labels that we put to our experiences—for example, judgments—that cause distress more than the thought or feeling itself. We will teach you how to mindfully label your thoughts in a way that doesn't cause more suffering.

"The sky is blue," "The rice is cooked," and "The table is made of wood" are examples of labeling with factual words. You can do the same thing with feelings, which so often get judged or invalidated by the labels we put on them. Those judgments unfortunately only enhance the very emotion you find uncomfortable. Examples of non-judgmental labeling are "I feel sadness," "I feel tears running down my cheeks," "My stomach feels hollow," "My shoulders are tense," and "I am hunched over." These labels are all facts that are difficult to argue with. Put into words only that which you notice in the moment. Don't add your own commentary or judgments to the experience.

In the earlier example of sitting on a park bench, you might notice a woman in sneakers, red shorts, and a blue top jogging past you. Labeling the experience would go like this: *A woman wearing running sneakers, red shorts, and a blue top is jogging past me.* Adding *I think she's late for work, She must be worried about her weight, She should be on a diet,* or *She's wearing ugly shorts* would be your own editorial, assumption, judgment, and conclusion, not necessarily anything that others observing the same event would think about. Others would, however, agree that she was jogging and wearing the clothes as you describe. Certainly it's possible that your assumptions and conclusions are correct, but without knowing any more about the jogger, all we want you to describe is what you can notice using your senses and sticking to the facts.

The practice of labeling can be invaluable in dealing with emotions. Consider the example of anxiety and panic. Many people fall into this type of rut or habitual thinking as they experience anxiety: *I'm getting anxious. I hate this anxiety. I can't believe I'm so anxious. I am anxious again. This is awful! I can't control it. When will this end? I hate this so much. What is wrong with me?* And the thinking can go on and on. If you pay attention as the chain of thoughts continues, the anxiety increases. The alternative would be to notice and label the anxiety by sticking to the facts, which could look something like this: *I'm getting anxious. My heart is beating fast. My palms are sweating. I'm breathing more quickly. I feel dizzy. My thoughts are moving quickly. I feel hot.*

By noticing the anxiety and then labeling it (putting precise words to your experience), you let the anxiety run its course without increasing its intensity. Being able to notice and then label can also help keep you grounded in your experience so that you don't get swept away in the emotion and all of the thoughts that follow.

Use Your Words

Imagine coming across a flower that you have never seen before. You use the experience as an act of mindfulness and then put the following words to the experience: "The plant has alternately arranged leaves and is 10 centimeters long and 4 centimeters wide. The leaves vary in shape, ranging from straight to tear-shaped, with toothed or wavy margins. The flower is a four-petal bloom in the shape of a cup. The stigmas and stamens are yellow in color. It closes its petals at night." Now, an expert might recognize this as a pink primrose, but if you had no idea what it was, you would have done a fine job of describing what you saw. Saying "I see a beautiful, pink flower" is not labeling completely and adds the judgment "beautiful," and as such would not be consistent with mindful practice.

Thoughts Are Not Necessarily Facts

When it comes to awareness, labeling is paying attention and putting words to your internal experience. Let's say, for instance, that you're struggling with writing a report that's due tomorrow. You start to get a stomachache, and begin to sweat a little and worry that you are going to fail the class or get fired from your job. You try to get the report written, but you feel completely overwhelmed and hopeless, and say, "I just can't do this." What you have just said is a thought, not a fact. You may in fact be able to write the paper even if you think you can't. Labeling these thoughts and feelings would go something like this: *I have to write this report. I notice that I have become anxious about writing the paper. I notice that I have the thought that by not writing the paper, I will fail the class or get fired.* It's almost as if you were describing something outside of yourself, as if you were a researcher observing other people describing their experience.

> A young man with BPD who was studying at night school asked a classmate out on a date, and she said no. He concluded that she hated him, and the thought *That girl in my class hates me* became a fact in his head. Rather than recognize that this was just a thought he was having, he regarded as "fact" that the girl actually hated him. It turned out that she was shy, hadn't been asked out before, and didn't know what to say, so she said no. But the young man had turned his thought into a "fact." Using the skill of labeling, he might have thought, *I notice that when the girl said no, I had the thought that she hates me. I realize that it's just a thought and that I have no information to confirm that this is actually so.* You will notice that working with your mind in this way leaves you with some uncertainty. It is important to realize that while you may have some discomfort with uncertainty, in the end that type of uncertainty may be less painful and easier to tolerate, and have fewer negative consequences, than the assumptions that your mind will make. Remember, you can use noticing and labeling skills to tolerate uncertainty and remain open to the reality in front of you.

Like noticing, the practice of labeling will teach you about yourself and the way you think, and put you in greater control of your experience. Knowing that what you think is just a thought, knowing that wondering what will happen if you don't write the paper brings up the thought that you are going to fail the class or get fired doesn't mean it's going to happen. Remember, a thought is not always a fact.

Stick to the Facts

An important aspect of labeling is sticking to the facts and doing so without judging. We will talk about judging in the next section, and you will see that many of us judge much of the time. Judgments are shortcut ways of describing an experience, and generally others know what we mean. It may be obvious to say that when we judge something as good or bad, that's our perspective. We don't normally explicitly say so, however. For instance, you might as a friend, "Tell me about your meal," and receive the reply, "It was disgusting." You might decide not to order the meal. If the labeling skill of mindfulness were used, the reply might be "It was broccoli covered in blue cheese." Now it's possible that you would find it disgusting, but it's also possible that you love broccoli covered in blue cheese. The fact that someone else finds it disgusting doesn't make it so to you. It only makes it so to that person. Labeling clarifies our experiences in the world and makes them more accessible to us and the people with whom we want to communicate.

Mindfulness Practice: A Meal

The next time you eat a meal, do so mindfully. See if you can use the labeling skill throughout your meal. Begin by putting words to the experience of sitting at the table. Using labels and sticking to the facts, describe the chair you are sitting on, the plate in front of you, and the table setting. Next move on to the food on your plate, the smells that arise, and the taste and texture of your food. Do this quietly in your mind. Pay attention to the whole experience. When you find yourself distracted by things around you, bring your attention back to noticing and describing your experience during your meal.

■

Mindfulness Practice: A Flower

For two minutes, look at a flower. Can you label its scent, its colors, its petals, and the emotions you experience when you hold it? Take your time and look at the details. You may get distracted or bored, or notice judgments; if you do, bring your mind back to the flower and begin labeling again. It's okay to repeat your labels; the goal is to practice labeling and keep your mind on this one task.

■

Mindfulness Practice: A Worrisome Thought

Sit quietly in your mindful position in a comfortable spot. Think about something that you are worried about. Avoid choosing something that elicits significant worry or anxiety, but think about something that maybe rates at 4 or 5 on a scale from 1 to 10. Notice, and watch and label the anxiety (and other emotions) and thoughts that arise. Label what happens to your breathing, any tension in your muscles, or any other thoughts. Do this practice for three to four minutes or until your anxiety drops below 3. As you begin to practice with higher levels of anxiety, you want to notice until your level of anxiety drops below the level where it was when you began the practice. Try to do this practice every day.

■

Mindfulness Practice: An Emotion

For two minutes, sit mindfully and label an emotion. Begin by identifying the judgments that you have about this emotion. Next, replace your judgments with nonjudgmental labels. Notice how the emotion feels in your body and describe it. Try this with multiple emotions, and write down your observations if you find that helpful. Do this same practice with the same emotion the next time you feel it. When you label the experience, notice whether the labels change or stay the same.

■

Mindfulness Practice: An Advertisement in a Magazine

Find an advertisement in a magazine that you find pleasant to look at. For two minutes, label what you see in the ad. Stick to the facts. Now, find an ad that you dislike (for instance, you may find the product or the models unpleasant to look at), and spend two minutes labeling that ad.

■

Nonjudgment

As we reviewed the skill of labeling, we began to talk about doing so nonjudgmentally. If you have consulted a therapist who used DBT with you, or if you have studied mindfulness or meditation, you will be familiar with this skill. Nonjudgment is central to the discipline of mindfulness and is a core component of DBT mindfulness. Being able to identify and let go of judgments is fundamental to practicing mindfulness, and a skill that needs to be practiced. Even if you consider yourself to be a nonjudgmental person, you may need to reconsider this. Most of us are not aware that we judge and that we live in a very judgmental world. If you don't see it, think about how politicians refer to each other, how tabloids portray celebrities, and how friends describe people they don't like. A nonjudgmental stance is essential to the practice of mindfulness.

For many of us, making judgments is habitual, and as with changing any habit, we must pay attention to when we make them. When you pay attention to judgments, you notice that they influence your thoughts, feelings, and behaviors. To develop this skill, start by simply noticing something, and do so without evaluating it; that is, stay away from words like "good" or "bad," "outstanding" or "horrible," and "should" or "shouldn't." Try to detach your opinions, approval, or disapproval from what is, and stick to the facts, as in the discussion of the skill of labeling. Before we get into the practice of a nonjudgment, we need to look more closely at judgments and how they function. The last thing you want to do is start judging your judging.

What's the Problem with Judgments?

So, what's the problem with judgments? One part of the answer is that, at times, there's no problem with them at all. However, often a judgmental stance around negative emotions can be both self-destructive and destructive to relationships. Automatically judging other people and ourselves means that we have made up our minds. This is also true of positive judgments, but generally positive judgments don't cause us much suffering. However, negative judgments or judgments that demonstrate a wish to change reality, such as that something "should" be different from how it is, often cause us a lot of suffering. In general, judgments leave little room for curiosity because you have already made up your mind. For people with BPD, judgments show up frequently and in many ways, especially in black-and-white thinking and judgment of emotions that feel intolerable. These judgments only make feelings more intense and intolerable, which often leads to destructive urges and behaviors.

Now if you say, "My emotions sometimes get me into trouble," that may be true, but simply judging your emotions as bad misses the fact that emotions are very important to the human experience. Judgments are often rapid and at times inaccurate interpretations of the world around us. Sometimes we need to use shorthand (judgments) in an effort to save time when we don't need to be exactly accurate, but if we do so when we are not paying attention, these judgments can cause a lot of suffering and lead back to a cycle of being thrown around by our emotions.

Emotions and Judgments

Our moods can permeate our thinking and therefore our judgments. For people with BPD, this is often the seed of mood-dependent behavior. Social psychologist Joseph Forgas (1999, 97) noted that people's "memories and judgments change with the color of their mood." Moreover, once you make a judgment, you are more likely to search for information that confirms or validates your judgment and ignores other important information. This can keep you stuck in the emotion. This phenomenon is called *confirmation bias*. This is particularly problematic once you consider both the rapid mood dysregulation in BPD and the often-chronic feelings of depression and anxiety. Here you can see how judgments can enhance uncomfortable emotions as well as narrow your thinking.

> Sonia, a thirty-eight-year-old woman with BPD and chronic thoughts of killing herself, stated that she could imagine living only if she could find a way to "stop feeling bad feelings." When she was asked to describe "bad feelings" nonjudgmentally, she shared that she did not want to feel sadness, fear, anger, guilt, or shame because these emotions made her miserable. At first glance, this makes sense. Of course, she didn't want to feel these feelings if they caused her distress; but how much of her distress was caused by the feelings themselves, and how much was caused by her judgment of her feelings as bad? If Sonia hadn't judged these feelings as bad, perhaps they would have felt more manageable and she could have used skills to change the intensity of these emotions. How much of her judgment made her filter out her

other feelings so that she saw only these so-called "bad emotions"? And how much of her distress was caused by the thoughts and behaviors that resulted from these judgments, which led to emotional suppression and avoidance?

As you learned before, suppressing emotions, which was one of the functions of Sonia's judgments, only makes emotions more intense. Sonia was constantly running from these emotions, which was exhausting. In fact, if we could have granted Sonia's request, it could have been quite dangerous, because she needed all of those emotions. Emotions have important and adaptive functions for communicating with and influencing others, organizing and motivating action, and validating our own experiences (Linehan 1993).

In general, our culture seems to judge feelings like joy, excitement, and love as "good" and feelings like anger, sadness, fear, guilt, and shame as "bad." We argue that it's not the feeling that is necessarily the problem, but the judgment that surrounds it. It's true that you may prefer some emotions to others, but the task is to begin to experience emotions nonjudgmentally, and watch and notice what you experience in the present moment. If you begin to experience an emotion, use your labeling skills to label the emotion as it is, describing how you feel it in your body, the content of your thoughts, and how these factors change over time. You will begin to see the emotion shift and ultimately decrease in intensity. This way, you won't feel that you have to run away from some feelings and desperately seek and hold on to others. All feelings will come and go.

Accept Reality as It Is

Now that you have learned about taking a nonjudgmental stance, it's important to spend some time on the concept of acceptance—that is, accepting reality as it is and doing so without judgment. In DBT this is called *radical acceptance*. Acceptance is one pole of the acceptance vs. change dialectic of DBT (Linehan 1993). For some people, accepting themselves and their lives as they are can be one of the hardest skills to master, and sometimes you have to accept things that are seemingly unjust or unfair, such as being hurt or treated badly. You may ask, "Why would I want to accept my life if I am unhappy with it?" This is an excellent question. When you can accept reality as it is, without judging it or fighting it, you can begin to look at how this reality developed, and perhaps what role you played in it or how you can change your response to it or your experience of it. Accepting things as they are doesn't mean agreeing with your reality or liking it; it means acknowledging that it is simply what it is. Accepting reality can profoundly influence your behavior, particularly when you are in distress. When you move into an accepting position, you begin to look at the situation from a different perspective. Remember that with acceptance can come pain and other intense emotions (nonacceptance can often help us avoid those feelings). There are skills that are very effective for managing intense emotions, but there are not many skills that help when you are in a state of nonacceptance. The challenge with practicing acceptance is that you may have to accept something over and over again, because you can easily slip back into a nonaccepting stance.

Consider this story about Jenna and how accepting reality nonjudgmentally could have helped her cope with her distress and maintain her self-respect.

Jenna had been dating her boyfriend for about a year. She was very much in love with him, but their relationship had been riddled with arguments and they had broken up a number of times. Jenna returned home one evening to find a note from her boyfriend that said he could no longer be with her. Jenna experienced this as a complete surprise. She began yelling and crying, sending more than twenty text messages and voice mails, alternating between angry and threatening and sad, replete with begging to get back together. Jenna felt desperate as she again heard that she was "too much to manage," so she became quite depressed and couldn't get out of bed. This situation was all too familiar to Jenna, and yet it always felt unjust and as if it came out of nowhere each time.

Where could acceptance have helped Jenna? Being able to step back and accept the situation in front of her could have helped Jenna to slow down, and while it would have been painful, she could have used some skills to prevent herself from sacrificing her self-respect by making so many calls and sending so many texts—which likely only added to the idea that she was "too much to manage" and made her feel even worse. Moreover, Jenna could have worked on accepting this pattern of relationships so that she could have begun to look at how she had contributed to her relationships ending this way, and she could have learned to pay attention to avoid repeating certain behaviors in her next relationship. Finally, as Jenna practiced acceptance, she could have begun to examine what she did have control over and could change, and what her boyfriend brought to the relationship that she couldn't change. In this situation, Jenna was challenged to practice acceptance (nonjudgmentally) of the situation, her boyfriend, and herself.

You may find practicing acceptance of yourself even more challenging. Many people with BPD who have difficulty managing emotions judge themselves quite harshly. They experience themselves as bad, ruined, toxic, unlovable, and undeserving. You will notice that those are all negative judgments, because people with BPD often struggle to make positive judgments about themselves. As we discussed, those negative judgments and nonacceptance lead to a lot of suffering. Developing self-compassion and acceptance is also a mindfulness practice. Sharon Salzberg (2008) has made popular an ancient form of meditation called *metta*, or *loving-kindness meditation*. Loving-kindness meditation teaches you to focus on seeing the goodness or positive attributes in others, rather than focusing on the negative or what makes those people challenging to be around. Salzberg believes that our suffering is connected to negative judgments. This doesn't mean that you ignore what may be challenging about others, but that you open your mind to compassion and focus on the positive. When you focus on others' negative aspects or your negative judgments about others, you suffer with feelings of anger, disappointment, dissatisfaction, bitterness, and hatred. This practice can further develop your skill of nonjudgment toward yourself and others.

You practice metta by sitting comfortably for at least three minutes, repeating a short phrase to yourself over and over again, and repeating similar phrases that "give" loving-kindness to others in your life to whom you want to send compassion or about whom you have negative judgments. There are many examples of phrases that you can repeat. Once you have practiced, you can use this as an informal practice when you find yourself suffering from negative judgments or emotions about yourself or others in your daily life. One example (ibid.) of a series of phrases you can use is:

May I be filled with loving-kindness.

May I be safe and free.

May I be peaceful and at ease.

May I be happy.

We encourage you to try this practice and observe how you feel when you are finished. You can replace "I" with the name of a person whom you are struggling with, or the name of someone you care about and want to send compassion to.

Here's one way to practice: when you notice a judgmental thought about yourself or someone in your daily life, say to yourself, *May you be free from suffering.* This interrupts the cycle of negative judgments and emotions that often follows a judgmental thought. We will return to this practice in later chapters.

Build Awareness

The first step in practicing nonjudgment is to commit to noticing your own judgments. Bringing your awareness to any behavior is the first step to changing that behavior. Sometimes simply the act of noticing the behavior can change it. It can be helpful to give yourself a signal (nonjudgmentally) that you have noticed a judgmental thought or statement. In some of our groups, members often point out judgments by ringing a bell or saying "Ding." We give other patients a hand counter that they can click every time they notice a judgmental thought. Once you have noticed a judgment, you can assess whether or not the judgment is useful. If it's not, try to rephrase your thought nonjudgmentally (sticking to the facts) and notice whether your emotional experience changes. Remember that judgments are not inherently problematic, so don't judge them as so.

Mindfulness Practice: Pain or Discomfort

For three minutes, identify an area of pain or discomfort (muscle tightness, headache, and so on) in your body. Look specifically for discomfort that you feel particularly judgmental about. As you watch and notice your thoughts, find the judgmental thoughts that arise within you, and using your labeling skills and without judgment, reframe your judgmental thoughts into ones that are free of judgment and fact based.

■

Mindfulness Practice: Political View

Spend thirty minutes to an hour watching a news station or reading a newspaper that holds a very different political view than you do. If you consider yourself liberal, read or watch something conservative; if you consider yourself conservative, watch or read something liberal. Notice your judgments as they arise when you watch or read. See if you can transform some of these thoughts into nonjudgmental descriptions.

■

One Thing in the Moment

The next skill that is fundamental to how you practice mindfulness is learning to do one thing in the moment. Marsha Linehan (1993) calls this doing things "one-mindfully." When you are reading, just read; when you are talking with a friend, focus only on the conversation; when you are eating, eat; when you are walking, just walk. Most of us tend to do many other things, like reading the paper, checking e-mail, or answering texts, at the same time that we are walking, eating, or talking to a friend. Doing one thing in the moment is a powerful and useful, yet challenging, skill that is particularly relevant in our fast-moving culture filled with multitasking.

The key here is to let go of all attempts to do many things at once. This includes letting go of all the thoughts racing around in your mind and putting your mind and body to the task of doing just one thing in the moment. This can feel impossible when you are facing multiple deadlines, and you will find it easier some days than others. Initially, doing one thing in the moment might feel as if you are slowing down too much and won't get anything done, but you may find that whatever you choose to do, in the end you will get it done more effectively and efficiently. You may even be able to decrease your level of stress and increase your sense of mastery. The ancients knew this. In the first century BCE, a Syrian slave who became a writer, Publilius Syrus, wrote: "To do two things at once is to do neither."

Doing one thing in the moment works best if you practice throwing yourself completely into what it is that you are doing. The trick here is to let go of self-judgments and self-consciousness, and become one with the activity. What you are doing in that moment is all that matters. Actors, dancers, and athletes tend to be good at this skill. Imagine an actor, dancer, or athlete thinking about needing to prepare dinner or do laundry during a performance or game. Most wouldn't do their best, because they would be distracted by their thoughts. Skilled actors fully participate in the performance without getting caught up in their thoughts or worrying about other things. They are present in the moment that is in front of them. Full participation in something often quiets the mind, and many people find that fully participating in an activity brings joy and some peace.

The formal practice of mindfulness has its roots in Buddhism, which has a way of making a point through short stories known as "Zen shorts." Here's a nice Zen short that captures what it means to participate completely in one moment with intention (Thích Nhất Hạnh. 1995, 14):

> One day the Buddha was speaking to a prince. The prince asked him, "What do you and your monks do in your monastery?"
>
> The Buddha said, "We sit and we walk and we eat."
>
> The prince said, "Well, how are you and your monks different from me and my people? For we do all those things as well."
>
> The Buddha responded, "When we sit, we know we are sitting. When we walk, we know we are walking. When we eat, we know we are eating."

By participating completely in each moment and with awareness, we move away from the stresses of our lives and learn to recognize that this is where we are and that we are okay right now. This doesn't mean that we neglect other things in our lives, but that we live in the moment, not in the past or in predicting the future. Do what you are doing and nothing else.

Multitasking: Deluding Yourself

Increased stress and loss of time—what else is a consequence of multitasking? Christine Rosen (2008) cites the work of psychologist Russell Poldrack, who found that "multitasking adversely affects how you learn. Even if you learn while multitasking, that learning is less flexible and more specialized, so you cannot retrieve the information as easily."

When we talk about multitasking, we are really talking about what happens when we are paying attention, how we switch our attention between tasks, and the judgment that we use in deciding what we should pay attention to. Many very successful people achieved success in their fields because of their capacity to focus their attention on the task at hand. The famous scientist and genius Isaac Newton noted that he attributed his discoveries "more to patient attention than to any other talent." To summarize, multitasking:

- is less efficient, because the act of multitasking wastes time in switching from one focus to another and then back again;

- produces stress, something that's best minimized when you have BPD;

- makes it more difficult for you to learn.

Doing one thing in the moment is difficult and demands a lot of practice, but the payoff is worth it. Short practices each day can quiet the mind significantly, and you can do this practice anywhere. The breath is a wonderful anchor for a busy mind because it's always with you, so noticing your breath is a common way to practice focusing on one thing in the moment.

In Times of Mental Chaos, Tackle One Problem at a Time

Some people with BPD come looking for help with reducing the chaos of a mind that's spinning with troubles. They notice feeling overwhelmed and anxious. One of the risks of high anxiety is over-simplifying situations and reverting to all-or-nothing thinking. Alternatively anxiety can lead to shutting down and making impulsive decisions. These reactions usually result in even more problems and rarely end up solving the situation you are trying to deal with.

Sometimes when your mind gets going very fast, you'll notice that you cannot even identify what the problem is, let alone try to solve it. Moments like these can be an opportunity to step back, watch, and notice without judgment that your mind is racing at a thousand miles an hour; and practice doing one thing by choosing to focus on one thing in the moment.

> Tim, a forty-seven-year-old man with BPD, was regularly on the verge of quitting things: his job, a relationship, small tasks around the house, and so on. His problems seemed too big, and each time he thought about what he needed to do, his thoughts cascaded into a pool of insurmountable challenges that left him drowning in misery and ready to give up. As Tim began to practice, he started to see the benefit and wisdom of doing one thing in the moment, and he began to make headway with organizing, prioritizing, and completing tasks, and doing so with much less anxiety.

Mindfulness Practice: Eat Breakfast

When you have breakfast tomorrow, simply sit and eat your breakfast. Don't read the paper, look at your e-mail, or read the cereal box. Notice your experience. Notice when you become distracted by urges to do other things, and bring yourself back to the full experience of eating breakfast (experiencing the tasks, smells, temperature, and so on).

■

Mindfulness Practice: Drive

The next time you go for a drive, don't turn on the radio or talk on your cell phone. Simply drive. Pay attention to the movements you do in order to drive (braking and using the gas); notice the other cars on the road and the places you pass as you drive. When your mind becomes distracted, bring it back to the task of driving.

■

Mindfulness Practice: Watch Television

These days many people watch TV while checking e-mail or playing on their smartphones. The next time you want to watch your favorite show or sporting event, simply watch the show without engaging in other activities simultaneously. Turn off your computer and cell phone, and just watch.

■

Mindfulness Practice: Wash Dishes

Washing dishes can be an excellent way to practice your mindfulness skills. The task here is to participate completely in washing your dishes and only that. Notice the changing temperature of the water, the differing textures, the soap, and the bubbles. As your mind wanders to other thoughts, bring it back to this one experience of washing the dishes. Approach this task as if you have never washed dishes before.

■

Mindfulness Practice: Make a List

In the morning make a list of things that you need to complete that day. Rank them in order of priority. Do not start the second item until you have finished the first. If you do not complete the list on the first day, continue to follow the list the next day until you have completed each task.

■

Do What the Situation Calls For

As we discussed in chapter 1, people with BPD often get caught up in being "right" instead of effective, which can be very destructive in relationships and can result in sacrificing your self-respect to prove a point. The final concept of how you practice mindfulness is to learn to do what the situation in front of you calls for, or be aware of when you are choosing not to. Marsha Linehan (1993) calls this "effectiveness." This skill goes hand in hand with the other mindfulness skills, because the task is to learn to step back and assess your reaction or response to a situation, and be aware of your own thoughts, feelings, and judgments. We are asking you to step back from the idea of being right, and think more about what works when you respond to a situation and what would have the most long-term benefits. It is here that our emotions around being right can cloud our judgment, and in those situations, you and your relationships can suffer. Remember, thoughts such as *I deserve* or that things *should* or *shouldn't be* a certain way can be helpful indicators that you are getting stuck in being right and are not doing what the situation calls for.

There are many daily activities that will challenge you to use this skill. Imagine going out to dinner to a Chinese restaurant with a group of friends whom you are just getting to know. Very quickly you realize that everyone at the table can use chopsticks with ease. You feel embarrassed that you can't do so, and begin thinking that you "should" be able to eat like everyone else and that they will judge you for using a fork. You try to manage chopsticks, but realize that you will not be able to eat dinner that way. Doing what the situation calls for is using your fork despite your feelings about being different from your friends.

Driving is another wonderful opportunity to practice this skill. Have you ever been pulled over by a police officer for speeding when you were sure that other cars around you were going the same speed or faster? This happens all of the time, because only one person can get pulled over at a time. You may have the urge to argue with the officer about this fact, and you may be correct in your assessment. However, if you begin to argue, you will likely make your situation worse, and by expressing anger at the officer you could end up with a worse consequence. Although you may be right, accepting the consequence is what the situation calls for.

For people with BPD, this skill can be vital in learning to maintain relationships and not suffer with intolerable anger and behaviors that go against your personal values. So often, the chronic sense of being wronged by others makes it nearly impossible to forgive others' small indiscretions or mistakes, and as a result, people with BPD experience painful feelings of anger, rage, resentment, and hopelessness.

Lindsay, a thirty-year-old with BPD who was slowly and effectively rebuilding a relationship with her father after a difficult childhood, became enraged when her father wrongly accused her of buying the wrong brand of detergent for her mother and asked her to return it to the store. Lindsay quickly became enraged, because her mother had requested the very detergent that she had purchased. Lindsay responded to her father with a number of expletives and in a particular way that she knew would enrage him, and then she left the house.

A kind person, Lindsay didn't believe in treating people this way. As she walked along her street, her anger began to build and she felt increasingly out of control. She was afraid of the intensity of her anger as she thought of all of the ways in which her family had wronged her, how they had destroyed her life, and how in turn she had destroyed the lives of others.

This was no longer about detergent. Lindsay began to feel increasingly overtaken by her emotions, and the magnitude of her pain and suffering was intolerable as she started thinking that her life would always be like this and that others would always mistreat her and she would always mistreat others. With some help, Lindsay was able to take a step back and look at the situation. She noticed that she had lost sight of the initial problem of the detergent.

In this case, Lindsay was completely right: she had bought what her mother had asked for and been wrongly accused. However, she had also worked hard to rebuild a relationship with her dad. Most important, Lindsay was suffering the most by holding on to this anger and building resentment. So, Lindsay's therapist asked her, "Do you want to be right, or do you want to be effective and do what the situation calls for?" In moments like this, this is a difficult question to answer. After some time, Lindsay decided that holding on to her anger was causing her to suffer and that apologizing to her father for mistreating him, even if she was right and had been wrongly accused, was what the situation called and what would ultimately decrease her own suffering. Situations like this challenge you to use all of your mindfulness skills.

Mindfulness Practice: Past Behaviors

Think of a time when you found yourself being "right" instead of effective. What emotions got in the way? What would you do differently if you could go back and act effectively? How would the outcome have changed? How would your own internal experience have changed?

■

Mindfulness Practice: Family Members

Think of a time when someone in your family was clearly "wrong." Could there have been any benefit in letting go of the situation even if you were "right"?

■

In this chapter we reviewed and expanded on the core mindfulness skills of DBT. Remember that you must practice the skills you have just learned over and over again, with intention. Skilled mindfulness practitioners always return to the basics, so this chapter is an important one to return to.

In the next part of the book, we will look at specific symptoms of BPD and how you can use the mindfulness skills you have just learned to target these symptoms.

Part 3

The Lived Experience: Mindfulness as the Path to Freedom from Suffering

Chapter 5

Emotion Dysregulation

E motion dysregulation is at the core of BPD (Linehan 1993). In chapter 1 you learned the ways in which dialectical behavior therapy organizes the diagnostic symptoms of BPD, and we introduced additional symptoms that people with BPD report interfere with their lives. You will remember that emotion dysregulation includes emotional instability, mood reactivity, difficulties with anger, and "contagious" emotions, or extreme sensitivity to others' emotions. Mindfulness is extremely important for emotion dysregulation, because if you don't pay attention, you can quickly get dragged around by your emotions, which, as you know, powerfully influence your behavior. This chapter and the following chapters will teach you how to apply mindfulness skills to your BPD symptoms. Remember, there are always opportunities to practice mindfulness, so continue to think about how you can apply these skills to situations in your own life.

Emotional Instability, Reactivity, and Anger

Karen, a twenty-seven-year-old graduate student, has extreme difficulty with managing her mood and, in particular, her anger, which has had a severe impact on her relationships and her ability to complete tasks and meet her goals. Karen and her mother had worked hard to build their relationship, but Karen's mood reactivity continued to cause ruptures. One evening Karen's family held a dinner party. She was excited about the party, invited some of her own friends, and helped organize and set it up. Over dinner, Karen's mother and a number of guests began discussing the political issues in Israel. Knowledgeable and passionate about this topic, Karen entered into this debate, which soon got heated. Karen began yelling, firing off questions at her mother, and making comments like "How can you be so uneducated?" and "What gives you the right to say that?"

The guests and Karen's mother became quiet as the topic of conversation rapidly changed to Karen and her mother's relationship. Karen began swearing and got close to her mother, knocking over her own chair. As Karen became angrier, she lit into her mother: "Your political positions have screwed me up, and I will do everything in my power to make sure you don't screw anyone else up. You are a waste of a mother, and now your friends can see what you are really like." Furious, Karen left the house, leaving the guests rattled. She later told her mother that she had written apology notes to the guests; however, when her mother asked her friends about this, they said they had never received such notes. Karen reported that the guests must have lied to her mother.

Living with this much anger caused Karen tremendous suffering, and when we asked her what had gotten her so angry, the very question angered her, and she responded, "I don't know; it just happened."

Like Karen, people with BPD often feel that their emotions control them. What is particularly challenging is that the symptoms of emotional instability, mood reactivity, and difficulties with anger can easily feed off each other, becoming intertwined and creating a vicious cycle of emotional turmoil. You can see how Karen's mood was powerfully and rapidly triggered by her frustration at her mother and the topic of conversation, and ultimately led to uncontrollable anger. For Karen, the situation only seemed to get worse. Mindfulness skills will help you take control of these emotional ups and downs, and break the cycle of reactivity and anger.

Applying Mindfulness Skills to Emotion Dysregulation

So, how do you use mindfulness to work with emotion dysregulation and anger? In chapter 4 you learned some basic mindfulness skills, but where do you begin and how do you apply them? What could Karen have done differently? First, it's important to remember that keeping up a formal practice is critical so that when you get intensely dysregulated, you can draw on the skills that you practiced when your emotions were not as intense. The more you practice mindfulness, the more you can control your emotions instead of allowing your emotions to control you. It's important to understand that practicing these skills when your emotions are at lower intensities will enable you to use these skills in moments of high distress.

Again, you can liken developing mindfulness to learning to drive: first you practice in an empty parking lot, and then you take the skills you learned in the parking lot to more intense and anxiety-provoking settings like residential streets, followed by main roads and then highways. Your driving skills begin to broaden, enabling you to handle more stressful and complex driving situations and weather conditions. Mindfulness practice should be similar. Start slow and quiet and then use it in more complex situations as you get more comfortable. This happens slowly over time. There is no formula predicting the number of times you will need to practice before you can use these skills in any moment.

You have already learned some basic formal mindfulness skills and practices. Commit to practicing the skills during different levels of emotional intensity, beginning at low levels and then trying them out in more stressful or emotionally challenging situations. As you learn how to apply mindfulness to your BPD symptoms, notice how each practice draws on the foundational skills. Practicing doing things with intention, watching and noticing, labeling, taking a nonjudgmental stance, doing one thing in the moment, and being effective will help you to increasingly use mindfulness in your daily life.

Mindfulness Practice: Notice and Label—RIDE THE WAVE

When you struggle with emotion dysregulation, it's often quite difficult to notice and label your emotions, even in moments when your emotions aren't that intense. Karen's anger rapidly intensified and got the better of her during dinner. People with BPD often feel that their emotions go from 0 to 60 in an instant, and figure out what happened when it's "too late." This can be a painful way to live. Using mindfulness to notice and label your emotions when they are not so intense, to become aware of when the intensity changes, and then to label your experience is vital to overcoming emotion dysregulation. In DBT this practice is known as being mindful of your current emotion (Linehan 1993). To help you understand the steps involved in this approach, we have developed the acronym RIDE THE WAVE:

1. **R**egister your body sensations.

2. **I**dentify your action urges.

3. **D**etermine the emotion.

4. **E**xpress to yourself nonjudgmentally.

5. **T**ake deep breaths.

6. **H**ands and body are open.

7. **E**stablish a grounded position.

8. **WAVE:** **W**atch **a**nd notice your emotion as if it were a *wave*.

These steps will help you increase your ability to notice and label your emotions and slow them down. Remember that just paying attention to your emotions can start to decrease the intensity. The more you practice this, the better you will get at it and the easier it will become. Since you are just learning this skill, we recommend practicing it at least once a day as an emotional check-in when you are feeling little to no distress. It's a practice in paying attention to your experience in a particular way.

The goal is to be able to use this skill during all levels of distress; however, when you are beginning this practice or in very emotionally intense situations, you will need to step back from the situation at hand by asking for a break and going to a different room or outside so that you are better able to focus on the practice and your experience. Again, this is a "muscle" that you are building, so practice this way of paying attention in your daily life. Once you do that, you will notice that in times of distress, you can easily reach for this type of mindful emotional check-in to slow yourself down. Remember, awareness of needing a break and asking for it is mindfulness. Here's how to use RIDE THE WAVE.

1. **Register your body sensations.** One of the functions of emotions is to give you information about your experience. One way to get that information is to pay attention to your body sensations; all emotions have body sensations that can be helpful clues in identifying emotions. For example, Karen might have been able to notice signs of anger, such as tightness or pressure in her chest; warmth in her face; or shoulder, back, or neck tension. Generally body sensations increase in intensity as the emotion increases in intensity. There is no specific body sensation that always goes with a specific emotion, but there are some common body sensations that people experience with certain emotions, and you can watch for them as you practice. As you pay more attention, you will get more familiar with your own body sensations and feelings that accompany your emotions. Here are some examples of

what you might experience, but we want you to develop your own labels and define your own experience:

■ *Anger: Chest and shoulder tension, a sense of pressure building up, warmth in your face, yelling*

■ *Fear: Butterflies in your stomach, shakiness, a pit in your stomach, a lump in your throat, urges to run or hide*

■ *Joy: Lightness in your body, a smile on your face, laughter*

■ *Love: Feeling warm toward others, a lightness in your step*

■ *Sadness: Heaviness, emptiness, hollowness, sluggishness, stillness, tears*

■ *Shame: Tightness all over your body, curling into yourself, feeling jittery or numb*

2. **Identify your action urges.** Emotions are accompanied by action urges that give you further information to help identify what you are feeling. Just because emotions have urges doesn't mean you have to act on them. Imagine if you acted on your every urge how much trouble you would find yourself in. As with body sensations, there are also some common action urges for emotions. Here are some examples:

■ *Anger: The action urge is to attack.*

■ *Fear: The action urge is to flee, freeze, or fight (you may know this as the "fight-or-flight" response).*

■ *Sadness: The action urge is to isolate and withdraw.*

■ *Shame or guilt: The action urge is to hide.*

3. **Determine the emotion.** Once you have identified the body sensations and the action urge, the next step is to name the emotion or emotions that you are experiencing. The act of naming the emotions can help you to feel more grounded in your experience and more in control. Not knowing what you are feeling can cause even more distress than the feeling itself.

4. **Express to yourself nonjudgmentally.** As we discussed previously, negative judgments can increase the intensity of your emotions, which can be a pitfall when you are being mindful of your emotional experience in the moment. The goal here is to express to yourself the emotion you are feeling and to do so nonjudgmentally; for example, *I am noticing anxiety* instead of *Oh God, I'm anxious, I shouldn't feel that way,* and *That's so stupid.* Using phrases such as *I am noticing* and *I feel an emotion* can be helpful. Remember that you are not your emotions and that your emotions won't last forever. When you say to yourself *I* am *anxious,* it can signal an inevitable permanency from which you might not imagine any escape.

5. **Take deep breaths.** As you RIDE THE WAVE, remember to breathe. Paying attention to your breath will help you to reduce the intensity of your emotions so that you won't move too quickly into action.

6. **Hands and body are open.** Keep your body in an open and grounded position. Make sure that your feet are on the ground, your arms are not crossed, and your hands are relaxed, not clinched. Try to relax your shoulders and the muscles around your eyes. Sit or stand up straight, and avoid hunching over.

7. **Establish a grounded position.** Place your feet firmly on the floor, and make sure that you can feel your sit bones making contact with whatever you are sitting on.

8. **Watch and notice your emotion as if it were a wave.** Now that you have paid close attention to your experience and identified the emotion, you can watch and notice the experience as if it were a wave. Remember that like a wave, the intensity will increase, peak, and then decline, like a wave crashing on the shore. As you watch the emotions decrease in intensity, you can elect to watch and notice for longer or shorter periods. As the emotional intensity decreases, you might find that you can begin to think more clearly, and identify ways to solve your problem and reconnect to your goals and values that often get lost during times of high emotional intensity.

RIDE THE WAVE increases awareness and gives you more control and choice about your actions and reactions. Once you have this awareness, you may need to use other mindfulness skills, such as accepting reality as it is or experiencing an intense emotion, like sadness, that you may have been avoiding. Karen may have needed to accept that not everyone at this dinner party would agree with her and that trying to change their opinions would only make the situation worse.

The best way to learn this skill is to set your intention to practice, and check in with yourself. Set a regular time. Find a quiet place and go through the acronym step by step. Learning to notice and label your emotional experience is invaluable and takes practice. When you get the hang of it, pay attention to times when you are unsure of what you are feeling, and RIDE THE WAVE. Be open and curious about what you notice, and let yourself experience it fully.

■

Mindfulness Practice: Use Nonanger with Others

Have you ever noticed that when people are most angry, they don't like to admit it? And many times people feel that venting about their anger helps diminish their anger. Feeding the anger you feel toward someone is rarely the solution; in fact it makes your situation worse, even if it feels satisfying in the moment. It can be like throwing gas on a flame. This is particularly problematic when it's done without awareness, and it's destructive to relationships. Many people also judge anger negatively, which you have also learned increases the intensity. While it may sound antithetical, the Dhammapada, an ancient Buddhist text, prescribes treating your anger with nonanger (Fronsdal 2005). This is not resignation; it's a way to decrease your suffering and loosen the grip that anger has on your life. Using nonanger with people will be the practice.

You will use this practice when you become mindful of feeling angry, frustrated, or irritated at someone in your life. You have already learned ways to identify anger in your body. Remember, you are labeling your anger without judgment. When the intensity of your anger begins to decrease, identify whom you are angry with. Next identify a way to practice nonanger toward that person. Acts of nonanger include giving a hug, buying a card, making a gift, helping out with a project, making the person a meal, or asking the person to coffee or lunch. Begin by practicing these activities when you notice feelings of irritation so that you will have plenty of practice when your anger is at a lower intensity. Practice curiosity about the other person's experience instead of anger. Let yourself fully experience your act of nonanger. You will find that this practice decreases your own suffering, which will ultimately help you maintain your relationships and be able to find resolutions to interpersonal conflicts.

■

Contagious Emotions

Most people with BPD are emotionally sensitive. Marsha Linehan (1993) uses a biosocial model to explain the development of BPD. In this model she describes a biological sensitivity combined with an invalidating environment as the two factors that lead to BPD. Linehan believes that people with BPD are born with emotional sensitivity, causing them to experience emotions more intensely, for a longer time, and with a slower return to baseline. Extreme emotional sensitivity is one of the things that leaves people with BPD feeling misunderstood, because other people in their lives cannot understand their deeply emotional experiences or reactions. They are often told that their reactions are "over the top," that they should "Let it go already," or that something is "not that big of a deal." Do these comments sound familiar? Because emotional sensitivity is understood to be biologically based, mindfulness will not get rid of emotional sensitivity but will help you to more effectively manage and accept that characteristic.

One of the challenges is that emotional sensitivity is not confined to your own experience; many times, it extends to the emotional experience of those around you. People with BPD can be extremely sensitive and aware of how the people around them are feeling. You can see how this can be problematic. Imagine being swept away by emotions that are not yours and that have little to do with what's happening in your life at that moment. Many people with BPD take on the emotions of those around them and, at times, confuse them with their own emotions.

One young woman described the feeling as being emotionally "porous." Imagine sitting in the waiting room at the doctor's office and noticing an anxious woman across the room shaking her leg. You might find that type of experience intolerable and begin to feel as anxious as the woman in the waiting room. This emotional arousal can quickly trigger confusion and distress as you search for the cause of this sudden-onset anxiety. This can be a dangerous quest to embark on, because your mind can quickly get away from you as it begins to search for things in your life (past or present) that cause you anxiety.

You can imagine that getting validation for such an experience from others would be challenging, because to many people, your anxiety makes no sense. This is further complicated by the fact that intense feelings may last for hours or even an entire day due to a slow return to emotional baseline. Does this sound familiar? Do you find it difficult to tolerate being around people who are very sad, anxious, or angry? Emotional sensitivity, contagion, and confusion can be very painful and can be harshly judged by others.

It's important to recognize that you might be sensitive to other's emotions and to do so without judgment. Being aware will help you to step back and make sense of what emotions belong to you and what emotions belong to someone else. By using the RIDE THE WAVE steps, you will identify your emotions. If you find yourself confused about why you are experiencing an emotion or if the intensity of the emotion doesn't seem to match the situation, you need to step back and assess where that emotion could have come from, and label it.

In the previous example, you would notice anxiety arising, and you might think, *I'm not in a situation that is anxiety provoking; however, I know that when I am around people who are very anxious, I often take on their anxiety. I am anxious because the woman across the waiting room is anxious.* This way of noticing and labeling allows you to take a step back from an emotion that belongs to someone else and not get caught up in it. Your practice is to get to know your own emotions and let other people have theirs.

The symptoms in emotion dysregulation are central to the diagnosis of BPD. Being mindful of your experience, noticing your emotions, learning to practice nonanger, and being aware of the impact that other people's emotions can have on you will help you break the painful cycle of emotional instability and reactivity.

Chapter 6

Interpersonal Dysregulation

Interpersonal dysregulation is another central feature in the suffering associated with BPD. You might have been called clingy, needy, or manipulative by the people closest to you, and these labels can be very hurtful. You might even feel that these things are true about you, or maybe others have told you that you are "too needy" so often that you begin to believe it. You will remember from chapter 1 that there are a number of symptoms of interpersonal dysregulation. We will focus on unstable relationships, fears of abandonment, and feeling misunderstood.

Charlie, a young woman with BPD, once described her experience with relationships in this way: "Sometimes, having borderline personality disorder feels like having slatted sunglasses. It seems like I see the world and my relationships in a completely different pattern and tint than everyone else does." Mindfulness can be a powerful tool to help you become aware of your own behavior patterns in relationships and begin to break some of the thinking patterns that may be the most destructive to your relationships.

One of the best-selling books about BPD is *I Hate You—Don't Leave Me: Understanding the Borderline Personality*, by Jerold Kreisman and Hal Straus (1989). The title captures the classic pattern of pushing away and pulling toward that many people with BPD and their loved ones experience in relationships. As we saw in chapter 1, these relationships are described in the *DSM* as "unstable and intense." Because the intensity and instability can lead to conflict, this in turn can lead to ending relationships, which can feel intolerable. If you have experienced this, you might then have come to the conclusion that no one will ever care and that you are destined to be lonely and misunderstood for the rest of your life.

Unstable Relationships

The relationships that people with BPD have with others who are close to them are characteristically unstable. In a study that compared the relationship quality of people with BPD to that of people without BPD, researchers found that people with BPD experienced more negative moods and greater changes in mood in the relationships than did those without BPD (Russell et al. 2007). In the same study, people with BPD reported feeling less dominant, more submissive, and quarrelsome in social interactions, as well as using more extreme behaviors than did people without BPD. Those in relationships with people with BPD often also experience the relationship as unstable. It is common to hear people talk about a relationship with a loved one with BPD as chaotic, confusing, filled with extremes (in both positive and negative ways), and chronically unpredictable.

> When we were sitting with a couple who were dealing with
> their relationship problem, John turned to his wife, Jacqui,
> who struggles with BPD, and told her, "You blow hot and cold.
> I never know where I stand with you." Jacqui recognized that
> this was true about herself, and she was also terrified that John
> would leave her.

Caroline, a twenty-three-year-old with BPD, came to the clinic feeling hopeless and suicidal due to chronic interpersonal conflict. Two years into her mindfulness practice, she shared with us her thoughts about her struggles with relationships:

> *A close friend of nearly six years decided not to talk to me*
> *anymore, citing my "clingy and suicidal behavior" as the reason.*

The more distance she put between us, the harder I pushed to be close to her again. I called her numerous times a day, even when it was clear that she was intentionally sending my calls to voice mail. I followed her around school obsessively, trying to talk to her about fixing the relationship. At that point, I was no longer in fear of her rejecting me and deciding to never talk to me again; I was actually watching it happen right in front of me. What was once a worried thought lurking in the back of my mind was now another loss, and a painful and unavoidable reality. The friendship was never resolved, and I graduated from high school having lost my other friends in similar ways.

The shame and anger from this experience were no longer just momentary emotions but had become a permanent state of mind with which I began college. I endured my entire freshman year still feeling an incredible amount of frustration and regret while trying to make new and lasting friendships. The pattern of "clingy behaviors" that were basically negative decisions continued, and I was asked to leave college. I could not seem to change my ineffective behaviors. To me, this reflected a personal shortcoming. I started acting on my insecurities about abandonment.

In treatment I exhibited similar aggressive and obsessive behaviors toward a hospital staff member. I would become furious when I felt she paid more attention to other patients, and this emotion manifested itself in verbal assaults. I would then obsessively and desperately try to fix the situation and relationship. I was making no progress. Again, as the person on the receiving end of my ineffective behavior set limits and took space, the cognitive distortions started firing: There must be something inherently awful and unfixable about me. *I became more angry and full of shame. I began having suicidal thoughts again, believing I was fated to fail at relationships for the rest of my life.*

With my reality so severely distorted, it was nearly impossible to see what my parents and my therapists had been telling me since the beginning. I couldn't see that my close friend of six years could have just been a seventeen-year-old girl who was too scared to serve as a confidant to a suicidal friend. Furthermore, by the time I sought treatment at age eighteen, my outlook on life was biased by the abandonment I had experienced. In hindsight and with mindfulness, I am able to see the causes of my suicidality and behaviors, and how I overcame them. The situations as they existed in reality were not unbearable, but the thoughts that shaped my view and the subsequent feelings certainly were.

Being able to realize that my thoughts can infringe on reality has become an important component in combating my unstable relationships and fears of abandonment. Mindfulness helps me to remember that these thoughts are just random neurons firing. Thoughts do not always equate to reality. I believe this inaccurate fusion of my subjective thoughts and objective reality has been the basis of most of my ineffective behaviors. Focusing on the present moment and not allowing my past experiences to bias my thoughts has produced effective results in my attempts to challenge my distortions and thus change some of my behaviors that end relationships.

Coming to terms with the more objective reasoning behind my friend's actions doesn't take away the excruciating pain of this lost relationship. I still find myself thinking about the fun and healthy relationships I used to have with my friends in high school, and how it feels like they were so unfairly cut short. I still hold in my mind the trauma of the rejection and the years of suffering I endured. However, I am no longer living in a constant state of unbearable emotions. Sometimes reality, as it exists, is still difficult and painful, but I find coping and acceptance much easier to achieve when I am free of distorted thoughts.

So how can you use mindfulness to target your interpersonal struggles? What can Caroline's observation and practice teach you?

Applying Mindfulness Skills in Unstable Relationships

Throughout this book we have looked at the painful consequences of being thrown around by your emotions. In BPD this often leads to mood-dependent behaviors, which you will recall means that when you are in a good mood, you can get almost anything done, and when you are in a bad mood, you either do nothing or, at times, make your situation worse.

Mood-Dependent Relationships

Not surprisingly, mood-dependent behaviors also show up in your relationships. We like to call what happens "mood-dependent relationships." Imagine your romantic interest standing next to a brick for two hours. Now imagine that you are in a very good mood for an hour and then in a very bad mood for an hour. You would likely agree that your perception of the brick is unlikely to change depending on how you feel during those two hours. Unlike your relationship with a brick, your relationship with the person you care about will be deeply influenced by your mood. You may find that if you are in a good mood, the other person can be the most wonderful person in the world, but if you are in a bad mood, the same person can be someone who suddenly irritates you, arouses your anger, or always lets you down.

At an extreme you may find yourself overidealizing at times and then, when your mood shifts rapidly, devaluing that same person. This is extremely painful for you and the other person. Because this is dependent on your mood, the other person's perspective or experience is often ignored. You can see how people in your life could be confused or even feel that you are unpredictable. When this pattern of overidealizing and devaluing persists and then things are going well in the relationship, the other person often has the feeling of anticipation that the "other shoe is about to drop." You would think that a partner would feel happy to be idealized, but when this way of interacting persists, many people feel that being on a pedestal and idealized means that there's only one way to go: down. So they live in fear of rapidly returning to the devalued position. Although we have all experienced our moods influencing how we feel about others, in BPD this can lead to very destructive behaviors, like physical fights, threatening, belittling, bullying, and insults.

How can you use mindfulness to deal with unstable relationships?

Mindfulness Practice: Get STABLE

The goal of this practice is twofold:

- To recognize how the state of your mood colors how you see the other person in the relationship

- To teach your mind that the other person and your mutual relationship are more than what you feel in the current moment

This is a practice in building awareness and gathering information. Approach this practice with curiosity. Remember that becoming aware of our behaviors and reactions is the first step. Find a time when you are calm, and think about five people you are close to. It can be particularly helpful to think of relationships that fluctuate with your mood. Try to identify times when you felt certain emotions, and whether those emotions colored how you felt about a person. Now go through the exercise of noticing and labeling your attributions, emotions, and judgments of each person. This practice will get your mind aware of and skilled in assessing the impact of your mood on relationships. In time, the goal is to continue to pay attention to this so that you become mindful in the moment when your mood may be prompting your behavior and thoughts about people in your life. We have developed the acronym STABLE to guide your information gathering. Here are the steps in the acronym STABLE:

1. **S**ad: Do you remember a time when you were sad about the relationship? How did you think about the

person? As you recall the situation, write down how you behaved, as well as your judgments and your emotions.

2. **Terrified:** Do you remember a time when you were terrified that the other person was going to abandon you? How did you think about the person? Again, recall and write down your behaviors, judgments, and emotions.

3. **Angry:** Recall a time when you were angry at the other person. Write down your behaviors, judgments, and emotions. Do you notice that you devalue the people whom you once idealized?

4. **Bored:** Do you remember a time when you were bored with the person? As in the previous steps, recall and write down your behaviors, judgments, and emotions.

5. **Love:** Do you remember a time when you were feeling intense love toward the other person? Once again, recall your behaviors, judgments, and emotions.

6. **Excited:** Do you remember a time when you were excited about the other person? You know the drill now. Write down how you behaved, your judgments, and your emotions.

Spend some time reviewing what you have written. What do you notice? Remember that the goal of this practice is to build awareness and pay attention to how your emotions affect your thoughts about important people in your life. Your responses may represent habits, so study what you have learned in this practice so that you can use this data as red flags when specific thoughts arise with people in your life. When the emotions and judgments show up, you can pause and recall that your thinking is being influenced by how you feel in the moment and that you are not seeing the totality of your relationship. It may be a signal to slow down and return to your RIDE THE WAVE skill to check in with how you are feeling before you act on any urges.

■

Mindfulness Practice: Your Typical Responses

We all have our typical responses to things in our lives. This is another exercise in developing your awareness of habitual or typical thoughts and behaviors that show up in your relationships. Take some time to reflect on the following questions. Again, this is important information gathering in the service of developing awareness. It's critical that you pay attention to your judgments. Many people with BPD have strong feelings, often including shame, about their ineffective thoughts. Feelings of shame and self-judgments lead to avoidance and prevent the building of awareness. Be gentle with yourself. Remember that with awareness, you can change the very responses that bring you feelings of shame and self-hatred, and gain control of relationship-destroying behaviors.

Take some time to think about and write down your typical behaviors and thoughts in the relationships that you find challenging.

■ *Typical behaviors in unstable relationships:* Perhaps you notice that when you are angry, your behavior includes starting or escalating verbal arguments, breaking things, quietly seething, shutting down, or insulting someone. Maybe when you are terrified that the other person will leave, you make multiple calls or send text messages several times a day. If you are sad, do you isolate, withdraw, or not do things with friends that would normally bring you pleasure?

■ *Typical thoughts* in *unstable relationships*: Again, the state of your mood can influence what you think, which then ties in to how you behave. If you are angry, you might think that the other person is horrible, or if you are terrified that the other person might leave, you might think that you are an awful person whom no one could ever love. When you are sad, you might think that you are always sad and that you are never going to feel better.

■

Mindfulness Practice: BEHAVE and THINK

The first two practices may seem simple enough, because we asked you to do them when you were calm. However, generally when you are calm, your relationships aren't blowing up. Remember that we are asking you to do many of these practices when you don't need them so that the necessary skills and awareness are in place when you do need them. Learning to drive in the middle of rush-hour traffic makes little sense, which is why you learn to drive on a quiet Sunday afternoon in a school parking lot. Similarly, practicing relational mindfulness when your mood is stable will help you the most in the long run, because you will build awareness and become familiar with the early signs or red flags that your mind is getting away from you.

But what can you do if you are in the middle of a relationship crisis right now? In the moment of conflict, you are going to target the two areas that destroy relationships: behaviors and thoughts. Remember, the more you practice mindfulness skills, the more effectively you will be able to practice them in the moment. Say that you are angry at your loved one and you are ready to blast the person. If you are about to behave in a relationship-destroying fashion (you identified your typical behaviors in the previous practice), mindfully BEHAVE:

1. **B**reathe and stay in this moment.

2. **E**xperience and label emotions as they arise.

3. **H**ear what the other person is saying and notice your judgments.

4. **A**pologize to the other person if you have not upheld your values.

5. **V**alidate (accept) that each of you may have a different point of view.

6. **E**xpand your awareness, taking in as many different aspects of the relationship as you can. Open your mind to positive, negative, and neutral memories and experiences.

If you find yourself thinking in a relationship-destroying fashion (you identified these typical thoughts in the previous practice), mindfully THINK. Take the previous situation in which you were angry at a loved one. In some cases you may not find yourself behaving in a destructive way, but rather *thinking* in a destructive way, such as *I am a terrible person* or *If my loved one cared about me, he wouldn't leave me alone.* Thinking can influence how we feel and behave, so you can see how your thoughts can also blow up relationships. When you notice your relationship-destroying thoughts, mindfully THINK:

1. **T**ake a breath to slow yourself down.

2. **H**old your hands open, palms facing upward.

3. Identify any cognitive distortions (review chapter 1).

4. You are **not** your thoughts.

5. Be **k**ind to yourself.

Practical tip: Remember to practice all the mindfulness skills when you don't need them so that they are in place when you do need them. One idea is to role-play with a good friend, a trusted teacher, or your therapist. Remember, the goal is to become aware of your relationship-destroying thoughts and behaviors so that you can use the mindfulness skills BEHAVE and THINK in the moment. As you practice, observe how your experience changes.

■

Fear of Abandonment

Fear of real or perceived abandonment causes tremendous suffering, because it leaves you living with a constant and enduring fear of loss. It's also one of the symptoms that throws your mind into a future that has not yet happened. Many people who fear abandonment miss the wonderful parts of their relationships that are happening in the present, because their minds have already jumped ahead to the "what ifs" of the future. The mind comes up with many ways to prevent this unknown future that is filled with imagined abandonment. One way is to push the other person away before he pushes you away, which can lead to devaluing of the other person after a period of overidealizing him. If you fear that you are going to be abandoned, there are a couple of possible outcomes:

The person is in fact going to leave you. You know this because the person has told you that he is going to leave you, or he acts in a way that tells you that he is going to leave—for instance, packing all of his belongings, never returning your calls, or starting to date someone else.

The person has no intention of leaving you. In this case and without any data, you imagine that the other person is going to leave you. Here, you suffer from a situation that is created in your mind, and you stick with the thought that tells you that people will always leave you. You might then begin to read meaning into the other person's behavior. For instance, you might decide that the person who hasn't called you has forgotten you.

How does fear of abandonment interfere with relationships? As Jane said one day in a therapy session:

> *The problem is I'm terrified of losing him. My mood swings and jealousy are just too much for him sometimes. He tells me that they don't make sense and that they are all in my mind. He does or says something, I take it the wrong way, and then everything spirals downhill from there. I seem to get stuck in that pattern; when I imagine him with another woman, I can't let go of the thought. I get so upset by what I believe to be true, and then I say mean and hurtful things to him. It all comes from my fear of losing him, and then when I say those things, I know that I will end up losing him—but I say them anyway.*

The Self-Fulfilling Prophecy

A common pattern in BPD relationships is that of the *self-fulfilling prophecy,* and it goes like this: you fear that a loved one is going to leave you, and this fear leads you to take action to prevent the other person from leaving. This behavior can involve actions that others see as "clingy" and "needy," meaning that you are constantly seeking reassurance that the other person is not going to leave, even after he has given you the reassurance that he won't. However, because you might have been left in previous relationships, you don't trust the reassurance, so you continue to take actions that test the other person's resolve to stay with you. The chronic nature of these behaviors drives people away, and then your worst fear comes true: the person leaves. When your loved one leaves, you then feel that people you trust and care about leave you, which leads you to draw the conclusion that everyone will leave. It's a "prophecy" in that you predict that it will happen, and it's "self-fulfilling" because you end up reacting to the prophecy by taking the very actions that cause it to come to fruition. What's so painful is that you end up causing the very thing you want to avoid.

Applying Mindfulness Skills for Fear of Abandonment

Because the fear of abandonment can quickly spiral into catastrophizing thoughts, you can use mindfulness to slow down. For many, the capacity to notice the early signs of this spiral is the place to begin. Again, as you build your mindfulness muscles, you will increasingly be able to notice the spiral beginning and not get caught up in it. Remember, for many people, fear is a fast-moving emotion that calls for reactions. With fear of abandonment, sometimes the fear is unwarranted, meaning that there's no evidence that the person is actually going to leave you, so you must notice if your fear fits the situation or is simply a worry that's not supported by evidence.

We have given you a number of acronyms in this chapter. These acronyms are meant to help you remember how to use these mindfulness skills in the moment.

Mindfulness Practice: Slow Down and Think SNAIL

The following acronym will guide you through the practice of slowing down when you notice fears of abandonment arising.

1. **Situate:** When you start to recognize the fear arising, find a place to be that's away from other distractions; for instance, go for a walk or go to a quiet place in your house.

2. **Notice:** Once you are still, notice the thought *This person is going to leave me.* Notice the emotions and thoughts that arise.

3. **Actions:** Notice the urge to act on your fear. Breathe and do not act on this urge. If it's helpful, don't change what you are doing. If you are sitting, remain sitting. If you are walking, continue walking until you notice the urge diminish. Consider turning off your cell phone and not using your computer for a few hours if these are ways that you tend to seek reassurance.

4. **Identify:** Identify the specific thoughts or emotions that are causing you to suffer.

5. **Label:** Label your thoughts as thoughts and emotions as emotions when they arise. Label what you know are the facts (*He hasn't called me in an hour*), and label what are assumptions and conclusions (*I am concluding that "Therefore he is going to leave me"*). Remember to do your best to stick to the facts even when your mind begins to produce many assumptions.

Using this mindfulness practice will not only slow you down and separate the facts from assumptions, but also likely prevent you from acting in ways that will push the other person away from you. As you have learned, this practice will continue to help you gain control over your thoughts and feelings, and do so in a way that helps you have more-fulfilling relationships and, importantly, maintain your self-respect.

■

Reinforcing Maladaptive Behavior

When Janet shared that she was ready to leave her emotionally unpredictable husband, Jeremy, who suffered from BPD, he threatened to kill himself and she felt trapped. "It's like emotional blackmail," she said. "I just can't leave him. I'd never forgive myself if he killed himself." The problem with Jeremy's behavior was that he had a persistent fear of abandonment and had worked out an effective way to get Janet to stay: he threatened to kill himself. They were both trapped in the relationship, with Jeremy unable to resolve his misery around abandonment and Janet unable to get out of an unhealthy relationship. Further, she was reinforcing his behavior by not bringing up how miserable she was in their relationship. In couples therapy, Jeremy agreed that on the one hand, he was terrified of being left and that on the other hand, he didn't want Janet to be with him merely out of her fear that he would kill himself otherwise. He wanted it to be "like when we first met, when she was with me because she loved me. She wasn't afraid of me then."

In this situation the task is to be aware as a couple. The pattern has to be recognized and articulated, and the reinforcing behaviors identified. In this case Jeremy's threat was reinforced by Janet's inability to leave, and Janet's need to stay with Jeremy was reinforced because it reduced her own fear that he would kill himself, something he said he would do if she left. Both Janet and Jeremy were suffering. Being mindfully aware and paying attention to your patterns is the first step to getting out of suffering; without that, you are simply repeating well-established behaviors that will perpetuate the cycle of fear of abandonment, anger, and shame.

Feeling Misunderstood

You may have told your therapists and others that you feel misunderstood, and in fact many people with BPD *are* misunderstood. Imagine trying to speak to someone who speaks only Chinese when you speak only English. It could be very frustrating for both of you. People with

BPD speak a very different emotional language, one with strong emotions and mood-dependent behaviors that others can have a hard time understanding. Thus, you may feel misunderstood, because on the most basic level, the people in your life truly do not understand you. Your language around emotions may feel like a foreign language to the people in your life. This is where things can get complicated. You might feel that the solution to this problem is to seek out people who understand you. Finding such people may help, but you also have to help the people who are in your life understand you.

> An emotional Aaron was talking about his relationship with his mother, and shared the following: "We simply are incapable of understanding one another, and any disagreement or argument results in our either yelling at each other, or angrily separating and going silent. I feel like she is trying to control me. She just doesn't get how hard I am trying."

Applying Mindfulness Skills When You Feel Misunderstood

Imagine again that you are talking with a person who speaks a foreign language. You have three choices:

- You can walk away and leave the person.

- You can teach the other person your language.

- You can learn to speak the other person's language.

In many circumstances, if you are close to the other person, simply walking away is not an option, so getting a better understanding of how the other person thinks and getting her to understand you is critical. Mindfulness can help.

Mindfulness Practice: GET ME and Get Curious

Feeling misunderstood is a familiar feeling for people with BPD. Some people feel that it's a chronic state that can be made worse by interactions with others or memories of such interactions. Feeling misunderstood, like many of the symptoms of interpersonal dysregulation, can spiral downward rapidly and lead the mind to filter in such a way as to call up more and more memories of times when you felt misunderstood. This cycle makes it difficult to pay attention to the problem and relationship at hand.

The following is another acronym to help you practice being mindful when you notice the feeling of being misunderstood arising. As with the other acronyms, it's important to practice these steps when the feelings are not as intense or not present at all, so that when the intensity increases, you can draw on your established skills. This acronym, GET ME, combines many of the mindfulness skills that you have already learned:

1. Ground yourself using mindful breathing (focus on your inhalation and your exhalation).

2. Express that you need space to figure out the misunderstanding.

3. Think about alternatives to your certainty about the other person's position.

4. Maintain an even manner by reminding yourself that everyone is doing the best they can.

5. Express yourself, clearly validating the other person's point of view while articulating yours.

■

Unstable relationships, fear of abandonment, and feeling misunderstood are misery-causing symptoms of BPD. Mindfulness can have a powerful impact on improving the quality of your relationships. You may start to notice that as you behave differently, so do the people you care about. Practicing mindfulness in relationships takes patience, because you are challenged to be aware of your own experience in the context of someone else's experience. As you develop the basic building blocks of mindfulness, you will find that it becomes increasingly easier to broaden your use of them to the complex situations that relationships often present.

Chapter 7

Behavioral Dysregulation

You learned in chapter 1 that behavioral dysregulation means that you use behaviors such as self-injury, suicidality, drugs and alcohol, disordered eating, unsafe sex, reckless driving, and other potentially life-threatening actions to regulate your emotions, especially in the context of relationships. Impulsivity and suicidal or self-injurious behaviors often show up when you are experiencing strong emotions, which can be another way in which you become dragged around by your emotions and thoughts. Getting pulled about in such a way can have serious consequences on your health and can result in your being hospitalized, being asked to leave school or getting fired from your job, and losing important relationships.

The problem is that in the moment, you don't think of consequences, because you have found a fast solution to decrease your pain. However, these kinds of behaviors keep you from reaching your long-term goals, which can make you feel more miserable and self-destructive as your life falls apart. You see how this can be a vicious cycle. Moreover, as we discussed previously, these behaviors provide short-term solutions to long-term problems, which you may even know at the time. This is another example of how getting caught up in strong emotions and the thoughts and urges associated with these behaviors leaves you trapped and feeling out of control.

So how can mindfulness help? Now that you are paying more attention to what's in your mind, you will discover that what precedes these behaviors, even the ones that you may feel are impulsive and just happen, are thoughts and feelings. You are beginning to learn what to do with your thoughts and how to avoid reacting. This may seem radical, but thoughts about self-injury and suicide are initially just thoughts. These types of thoughts are particularly challenging because they are intense and, for many, can be quite frightening and persistent. For some, they have a way of sticking around that causes a lot of distress. As powerful as the symptoms of behavioral dysregulation are, we want you to remember that initially, these symptoms start as thoughts, and thoughts are something that you can apply your mindfulness skills to. We will look at how you can use mindfulness skills to work on such thoughts before they turn into plans and actions.

Suicidality and Self-Injury

Tara, an eighteen-year-old woman with chronic and unrelenting suicidal thoughts and a long history of self-injury, was working with us in DBT. One day as Tara began learning about mindfulness, she shared the following:

> *Do you know what it's like to be afraid of your thoughts? I want to stop cutting and making suicide attempts, but when I begin thinking about suicide or when I have urges to cut, which is a lot of the time, I can't think about anything else. I am in it, and that's it. It's terrifying, I am my thoughts, and there's often no way out. Do you see why I'm anxious when I think about stopping? The worst is that I don't know when it will come up or if, in that moment, I will even care about not doing it. So, if I begin thinking about suicide or self-injury, I have to stop quickly or I will do something to hurt myself, but when I start telling myself to stop thinking, it makes it worse. Other times, I notice when my urges go up, like when I'm really angry, lonely, hopeless, disappointed, or just feel like I hate myself. Then I get sucked in so badly that it's all I want in the world. I stop thinking and then just do it, and right afterward, I feel better.*

Maria, a thirty-year-old woman, has a slightly different problem but one that's also common in BPD. Maria explained her experience with chronic suicidal thoughts like this:

I think about suicide all of the time; it doesn't matter what's going on. I know everything about suicide, and most of the time, it seems like the best option. It has been like this for years. It has become who I am, and it will never go away. It's a part of me, and honestly, I'm not sure what things would be like without it. It sounds really messed up, and for years, I argued that I should be able to just kill myself and that it was just meant to be, but now I'm not so sure. It's scary to think about life without suicide; it would just solve all my problems.

Suicidal and self-injurious behaviors are very problematic in BPD. People like Tara spend an enormous amount of energy trying to avoid thoughts about self-injury and suicide, and find themselves exhausted and unable to predict the thoughts that their minds will produce. Some have described this process as always playing defense against their minds. You can see the problem: eventually you run out of energy to defend, because your mind will continue to produce all kinds of thoughts. You have learned that suppressing thoughts can increase both the frequency and intensity of the very thoughts you want to stop thinking.

Other people, like Maria, have spent years thinking about suicide and have so much practice with that type of thinking that their brains produce thoughts of suicide as a way to solve their problems and strong emotions. The more you practice the thoughts and behaviors of self-injury and suicide, the more skilled you get at those behaviors and thinking those thoughts. While mindfulness won't provide as fast a solution as suicidal and self-injurious behaviors, it provides an opportunity to develop a new practice for dealing with such thoughts and for helping you to cut down on the behaviors associated with them.

Applying Mindfulness Skills for Suicidality and Self-Injury

Since mindfulness is about working with your mind, the following practices are designed to help you tackle these difficult symptoms before you act on them. Many people find that they go into automatic pilot when such thoughts begin and they simply cannot turn their attention elsewhere. The task is to identify and be aware of this kind of thinking early on, learn to be with such thoughts without taking action, and learn to turn your attention elsewhere when needed.

Mindfulness Practice: Get to Know Your "Self-Destructive Mind" and Ask Whether It's Helpful

We all have different modes of thinking that need to be defined and attended to so that we can catch our thinking before we get consumed by it and can't find our way out. Labeling a mode of thinking will help you step back and get some distance from your thoughts. It's another demonstration that you are not your thoughts. We would like for you to spend some time getting to know your self-destructive mind. If you struggle with suicide and self-injury, you will identify your "suicide mind" and "self-injury mind." Notice that there are no judgments attached, just the simple act of identifying the mode of mind.

If you are someone who gets easily caught up in these thoughts, you may want to do this practice with your therapist. If this is the case, begin to get to know a different state of mind for practice. For example, you can get to know your "nothing matters" mind, "no one likes me" mind, or "I'm not good enough" mind. Consider thoughts, emotions, and judgments that would give you clues that you are entering into this state of mind.

Do this practice as if you were a researcher gathering information about mind states. Keep a list of these clues that indicate you may be in these different states of mind, keep the list accessible as you develop this awareness, and spend some time learning them. Once you are satisfied with the list, identify some skills you can use when you notice that state of mind. Where would you like to be able to turn your attention? The goal of this practice is to identify your state of mind, take control, and determine whether this way of thinking is helpful. You want to keep doing it and decide whether you want to turn your attention elsewhere.

Once you get to know your different "minds," you can begin the practice. The practice goes as follows:

1. Notice and label your state of mind (for example, "self-injury" mind).

2. Ask yourself, *Is this way of thinking useful right now?* (answer yes or no).

3. If the answer to step 2 is yes, release your mind and let the thinking continue, knowing that this could make your situation worse.

4. If the answer to step 2 is no, identify alternative places to focus your mind. You may focus on a calming memory, some imagery, your long term goals, or perhaps a task or activity. Think about the image of picking up your mind as if you were picking up a brick and moving it elsewhere.

5. When your mind wanders back to the destructive thoughts, and it likely will for a while, label that state of mind that you are slipping back into and move your mind to a different thought or to a task to complete. Tasks that require thinking—such as doing crossword puzzles, playing logic games, or making a list of things you need to accomplish at home and

then doing them—can be useful. It can be helpful to say things to yourself like *There it goes again, Isn't that interesting that my mind went back there again,* or *"Self-injury" mind just came up as a solution to that problem.*

It's important to remember that this is a practice and one that takes a fair amount of energy. The more you practice, the more skilled you will become at stepping back from challenging self-destructive thinking and gaining the upper hand concerning where your mind goes.

■

Mindfulness Practice: Do You Inadvertently Practice Suicidal or Self-Injury Thoughts?

When you start paying attention, like Maria you may find that you have developed a habit involving suicidal or self-injury thoughts. Your attention is increasingly focused on these two things, not only in times of distress. It may feel as if these thoughts were always there, but it's more likely that you are paying more attention to them, that your mind is more captivated by them, making it more difficult to expand your awareness to all your other thoughts and experiences. When you develop such habits, you will likely engage in behaviors that support and continue them. To evaluate whether you practice such thinking, you can consider looking at ways that you might be perpetuating thoughts and behaviors around suicide and self-injury.

In times of distress, calmness, or boredom, what kinds of books do you read, what Internet sites do you visit, and what things do you write in your journal? What are the first thoughts you have when a problem arises? Do you buy items to use to hurt yourself, and keep them at home? Do you repeatedly visualize suicide or self-injury in your mind? Do you go over previous episodes again and again in your mind? Do you continue to engage in these behaviors? When you begin paying attention, you may find other ways that you practice having destructive thoughts. Most people who struggle with suicidal thoughts and behaviors and self-injury have developed habits that make giving up the behaviors even harder. So, once you are aware of your behaviors, how do you change your habits around them?

The good news is that you can change your habits. Remember that you learned that simply bringing your awareness to a behavior begins to change it. Make a list of your self-injury behaviors, suicide attempts, or both. For one week, make a commitment to pay attention and not engage in these behaviors. It's difficult to break habits, but you can use mindfulness to catch yourself engaging in one of these behaviors and stop yourself from continuing it. You can mindfully choose to do something that's not related to self-injury or suicide. For example, if you lie in bed and catch yourself using mental images about suicide or self-injury, see if you can replace those images with other ones that are unrelated to suicide or self-injury. The act of mindfulness is catching yourself in unwanted thoughts and returning your attention to your goal of abstaining from destructive behaviors. Pay attention to what happens to the quality of your thoughts when you begin to catch yourself and start practicing healthier behaviors.

■

Impulsivity

"I am impulsive. I just do things and don't seem to care about the consequences. There's nothing I can do about it, because there isn't time. If I want to do something, it's the only thing that matters. I have to do it." This may sound familiar to you. The problem with just saying or being told that you are merely impulsive is that it makes it seem as if there were nothing you could do about it. That's pretty scary. As the consequences of impulsive behaviors build, you might begin to feel pretty hopeless. So, if we look at the definition of impulsivity as acting on an impulse or urge instead of thinking about the action and consequence, you can begin to see how mindfulness can help this seemingly hopeless problem.

Remember that your mindfulness skills help you to slow down and pay attention to your thoughts without always reacting. Impulsive behaviors are another example of being thrown around by your emotions and urges. If you are working on DBT, you may use mindfulness skills to help you slow down so that you can look at the chain of events that leads to your behaviors.

Applying Mindfulness Skills to Impulsivity

Building your mindfulness skills so that you become less reactive will be the task ahead of you. Remember that with mindfulness, it's important to start building this muscle during formal practices, not in high-intensity situations. The practices we provide will be about working with urges rather than reacting. Your goal will be to avoid acting on strong urges and to get to know what happens to your thoughts in these moments. You will find that your skills will develop enough so that you can rely on them in real-life situations more and more. You are building your awareness of what happens in your mind when you are faced with a very strong urge to do something destructive.

Mindfulness Practice: The (Big) Urge to Swallow

This is an excellent practice to help you with impulsivity, because it is a practice that will elicit strong emotions and urges. Sit in a mindful position and set a timer for one and one-half to two minutes. Your task is to notice and not react to your urge to swallow. You will notice many urges as the saliva begins to pool in your mouth. It's okay to drool, but you must not give in to the urge to swallow. Notice what happens to your thoughts and how your urge gains intensity. Remember, you don't have to give in to this urge. At the end of the designated time, you may again swallow. It doesn't have to happen the moment your mind thinks of doing it. Take a few moments after this practice to observe your experience and how it may have changed from beginning to end.

■

Mindfulness Practice: Don't Move

Most people can identify the impulsive behaviors that get them in trouble; some happen in interpersonal situations, and others happen when you are alone. Now that you are developing awareness of your thoughts and urges around many things, you can try this practice. Sometimes the best thing to do is nothing at all; however, you have to be aware that this is what you need to do, and know how to do it. We taught you the RIDE THE WAVE steps in chapter 5, and this is a variation.

For this practice, identify an impulsive behavior that you engage in when you are alone (for example, self-injury, excessive online shopping, gambling, substance use, bingeing, purging, and so on). Make a commitment that the next time you notice the urge to engage in that behavior, you will do this practice. When you notice the urge (any intensity), you will commit to not moving. For many, lying on the floor or sitting in a chair or on the bed is helpful. We like the floor because it is literally grounding. The task is to commit to not getting up from whatever position you are in until the urge has subsided.

For some, this takes fifteen minutes, and for others, in the beginning, it takes an hour, sometimes longer. As you sit or lie down, focus your attention on your breath, and use your notice-and-label skills without reacting to the urge to engage in the behavior. You will find that you can ride out situations that used to feel impulsive, without doing anything at all.

■

Mindfulness Practice: Focus on Your Toes

You will first do this practice on your own in a formal way and then use it in everyday or emotionally intense situations. Consider doing the practice five to ten times before using this skill in the moment. For this practice you can sit or walk. If you are sitting, you will sit in a chair with your feet touching the floor.

Identify the feelings that often precede impulsive behaviors. Anger and jealousy are common, but think about the feelings that are most linked for you. For the sake of explaining the practice, we will use anger. As you sit or walk, begin to think about the last time that you were very angry, and notice the thoughts, feelings, and urges that arise. Breathe normally and pay particular attention to the urges that arise. When you feel that the intensity of your emotion is very high and you want to take action, shift your attention to your toes.

Begin by moving your toes; feel your toes against one another, or brushing against your socks or the inside of your shoes. Keep your attention on your toes, shifting your weight while you are seated or as you walk. If you are sitting, you may get up and walk around, as long as you keep your attention on your toes and feet. When your mind wanders back to your urges and emotions, ground your attention back on your toes. Continue to focus on your toes until you notice your emotions and urges diminishing. When this happens, begin to smile at how you have taken control of these emotions and how you can now approach the situation with a clear mind.

Once you become skilled at this practice, you can use it anywhere. Imagine getting in a fight with someone you care about and having the urge to yell at or hit the person. You will become familiar with the sensations of the feelings and urges increasing, and in those moments, instead of acting on an impulse, you will turn your attention to your toes, feel them on the ground, slow yourself down, and remember that you can walk away and get space from the situation instead of acting on impulse. You may notice some judgment arise, but we often forget that we can leave a situation without acting on an urge. Awareness of your toes and feet is not only grounding, but also a reminder that you can use this method to leave a potentially dangerous and consequence-laden situation.

■

Remember that you can try out the practices in this chapter and modify them after you have enough practice with them. Approach each practice with a beginner's mind, knowing that your experience may be different with each practice. Pay attention to when the practices seem to be more or less effective, or more or less challenging with your symptoms of behavioral dysregulation, and remember to return to these practices over and over again.

Chapter 8

Cognitive Dysregulation

Many people with BPD struggle with symptoms of cognitive dysregulation. In this chapter we will focus on the two most common cognitive symptoms: dissociation and paranoid thinking. Cognitive dysregulation in BPD means that a person has brief, nonpsychotic forms of distorted thinking. Cognitive dysregulation includes *dissociation*, which is when there is a lack of connection among your feelings, thoughts, memories, behaviors, and sense of self. Two forms of dissociation are *derealization*, which is the feeling that everything around you seems unreal and *depersonalization*, which is the feeling that you yourself are not real. The difference between the cognitive dysregulation in BPD and the disordered thinking in psychotic disorders, like schizophrenia, is that in BPD, the dysregulation tends to be brought on by stressful situations and the thinking distortion usually clears up when the stress is reduced.

Mindfulness skills can help you practice ways to remain grounded and try to redirect your mind when it begins moving in a direction that separates you from reality. This can be particularly challenging, because the mind often strays from reality during times of high emotional intensity and pain.

Dissociative Symptoms

Dissociative symptoms occur in about two-thirds of people with BPD (Ross 2007). Most studies of dissociation in BPD have reported that BPD patients have higher levels of dissociation than do people without psychiatric illness. This might not be surprising, but people with BPD have more dissociation than do people with every other psychiatric diagnosis other than dissociative identity disorder (Zanarini et al. 2000; Simeon et al. 2003). The most severe level of dissociation was reported when stress levels were perceived to be high (Stiglmayr et al. 2008). Finally, dissociation in BPD is more common if you also have other psychiatric diagnoses, like PTSD, substance abuse, *and* frequent self-injury behavior (Shearer 1994). Dissociation is also far more common in people with BPD who have been witness to or experienced violence, who have had inconsistent treatment by a caregiver, or who have been sexually assaulted in adulthood (Zanarini et al. 2000).

Kathryn is a twenty-nine-year-old artist with BPD. She describes her experience with dissociation like this:

Dissociation leaves me feeling numb, strange, and disconnected from everything. I feel like I'm just going through the motions of life without actually being me; rather I'm what I imagine a robot would be. During these episodes is when I cut myself, which can help bring me back, but then when I try to remember what happened, I can't. My memory just goes, and I can lose minutes or even hours of my day. I think that dissociation is a way for me to escape painful memories and feelings. Some people say I'm masking [hiding emotions], and there are times when I am aware of doing so, but most of the time, I am not.

Sometimes when I am going out and mixing with people, I don't feel that I am really "there"; it's like I'm watching myself through a mirror. I see that this person who is being happy, smiling, and having fun isn't really me; it's a mask, an act. The real me is locked behind the glass. None of it feels real, and anything that does feel real hurts, triggering a vicious cycle of more paranoia, self-harm, and so on. I am not sure when I will come back from this place or even if I will, and sometimes I'm not even sure I want to, because reality just feels like something I'm too scared to face at the moment.

Applying Mindfulness Skills to Dissociative Symptoms

Grounding is a skill that you can use to reduce dissociation. Grounding exercises involve the use of external sensations to reconnect with the world and to the present moment, and in this way, grounding is a form of mindfulness (Linehan 1993). Grounding challenges you to build awareness of your early signs of dissociation and work with your mind to remain present so that your mind doesn't take you back in time or away from the reality in front of you. You can use all of your five senses—smell, taste, touch, sight, and sound—to ground. One very powerful technique is the use of temperature—in particular, cold sensations.

Mindfulness Practice: Ice Diving

In our clinic, people who are struggling with getting grounded prepare a bowl of ice water and dunk their faces in it, concentrating on the temperature against their skin. This practice has the added physiological benefit of activating the dive reflex. While most strongly expressed in marine mammals, the dive reflex is also present in humans and is most strongly triggered when we submerge our faces in ice water. The dive reflex then slows down our breathing and our heart rate, essentially calming our physiology from the inside. You can see how this could be helpful during a panic attack.

Other exercises include listening to loud music, biting into a lemon, and smelling a scented lotion. The sensations these activities produce are powerful and can bring you back quickly to the present moment.

■

Mindfulness Practice: Grounding Mindfulness Kit

If you are prone to dissociation, try making a grounding mindfulness kit that you will carry with you. Identify strong sensations that work for you so that you can determine what to put in your kit. Some of these tools were introduced earlier in the book. Experiment with the following items when you are feeling grounded, and then choose ones to try when you notice early signs of dissociation:

- *Taste: Place in your mouth a piece of gum or hard candy that has very strong flavors. Strong mints or cinnamon-flavored, or sour candies work best. Savor the taste.*

- *Temperature: Use something cold. Hold ice cubes in your hand until they melt, suck on ice cubes, put ice on your wrists or under your eyes, stand on ice cubes, or put them in your socks. Keep cold fruit in your freezer; hold a frozen orange or eat frozen grapes. Put a cold cloth on the back of your neck, on your chest, or over your eyes. Run your hands under cold water, or splash cold water on your face.*

- *Smell: Find a scented lotion, a small bottle of perfume, or an essential oil. Try different scents; many people like to use lavender, while others like to carry scents that are comforting and familiar, like a loved one's perfume. Some people find that the scent of dryer sheets is particularly effective.*

- *Sight: Grounding using your sight can be helpful. Pick a category, such as shape, color, or even "first letter." Then look around and, in your mind, label each item that you see that fits in that category. For example, you might pick things that are blue. You would then look around and say to yourself, "I see a blue box, a woman wearing blue socks, a blue street sign." Each time, remind yourself and your brain that you are directing the experience by saying I see. When you have identified all of the blue items, choose another color. Do this for at least ten minutes. This gets your brain grounded in the physical environment around you. Keep bringing your attention back to this task of identifying.*

- *Sounds: Do you have music that you can listen to that you know will snap you back to the here and now? Identify different songs that help, and make a grounding mix on your iPod or MP3 player.*

- *Touch: Notice what's around you and where you are. Feel the cloth of your shirt or the fabric on your dress or pants. Reach down and touch things that are nearby in your environment and, in your mind, label the texture: This is smooth, rough, soft, hard. Lie down on the floor and feel different parts of your body pressing against the floor. Notice and label the changes as you inhale and exhale.*

Your task is to pay attention to the things that help you, and then as you begin to notice that you are dissociating, use your kit to practice grounding yourself. Part of using grounding is learning to pay attention to your own early signs of dissociation. Your therapist, friends, and family may be able to point out some early signs that they can see. Bring your noticing skills to this practice. Notice whether you feel sensations in your body like tingling, changes in vision, slowed thinking, heaviness, or difficulty moving quickly. If you are in DBT, completing a detailed chain analysis of the times when you have dissociated, and sharing the chain of events with your therapist, can be an effective way to gather this information.

It's important to do your best to commit to your grounding practice and keep practicing. It can be exhausting and take time, sometimes up to an hour, especially when you are learning. After grounding, use focusing on your breath to fully reconnect. If you can figure out what made you vulnerable to your dissociation, you will be able to pay better attention to moments that put you at risk. Therefore you will be better prepared to deal with future situations.

■

Paranoid Thoughts

Paranoid thoughts are thoughts of a suspicious nature in which you might believe, without much evidence, that something is not right with you, that others are out to get you, or that another's intentions are evil. Paranoid thoughts are considered to be psychotic in nature, and in BPD, unlike in major psychotic illnesses like schizophrenia, the psychotic thoughts tend to last minutes to hours, rather than days or weeks, and are often prompted by stress, many times of an interpersonal nature.

Barry is a twenty-three-year-old with BPD who has been in therapy for many years and has recognized that his paranoid thoughts have led to difficulty in getting close to people. This is problematic because Barry very much wants to have close relationships:

These thoughts occur at times when I am stressed out or am getting too close to someone. I get the feeling that the other person is mad at me or is intentionally trying to make me angry or feel guilty, and that's mostly when I cut or dissociate. It's hard to explain; I just know that that's how it is. Then I blame myself for getting so close to someone or for having trusted the person. I then feel that I can trust no one and that I should never get close to anyone, as if everyone I could ever get close to would do the same thing because I deserve it.

During these episodes of paranoia, I worry about what people think about me, and feel that there's something about me that causes people to hate me, that I don't deserve to be loved, and that the world would be better off without me. I get very certain about everything. Even when my therapist asks if there are other possible reasons why someone might have done something, all I can think of is the worst possible reason, imagining that what they want to do is to either hurt me or take advantage of me.

So, how can mindfulness help?

Applying Mindfulness Skills to Paranoid Thoughts

As we mentioned earlier, paranoia is a form of psychosis, and historically this symptom was treated with antipsychotic medication. Until more recently, people felt that mindfulness and meditation would not be an effective treatment for psychosis. However, in a recent study (Chadwick et al. 2009), twenty-two participants with distressing psychotic experiences were assigned to either group-based mindfulness training or a waiting list for mindfulness therapy. The mindfulness group attended twice-weekly mindfulness sessions and used meditation CDs at home for five weeks, and when the sessions ended, they practiced mindfulness at home for another five weeks. After this relatively short intervention, participants who practiced mindfulness found that there was a reduction in thoughts and images, and an improved ability to be mindful of the paranoid thoughts and images. Because paranoia can be a distressing symptom in psychotic disorders as well as in BPD, this study provides further evidence that mindfulness can be an effective tool in attending to and managing this difficult symptom.

Another way to think about it is that paranoia is a form of judgment. You are deciding that something or someone does not have good intentions, or that people are intentionally trying to harm you. You have already learned a number of different ways to take a mindful and nonjudgmental stance. The following are some ways that you can use the many basic building blocks of mindfulness that you have learned already to deal with your paranoia.

Mindfulness Practice: Your Top Five

When most people pay attention to their paranoid thoughts, they find that their minds produce the same or similar thoughts over and over again. Many people can find a few variations of the same five or ten thoughts. This is, in fact, a good thing, because it will help enable you to identify these paranoid thoughts quickly and categorize them. These thoughts are often judgmental, black and white, catastrophizing, or very confusing. Remember, these are just thoughts that your mind produces, and you are building awareness so that the thoughts no longer sweep you away. It's vital that you develop awareness of these thoughts so that you can catch them in the moment.

You might want to keep a small notebook with you and, when you notice a paranoid thought, write it down under one of the categories. Here are some common categories: thinking that others are intentionally causing you pain or harm, that people are looking at you and judging you, that others can know what is in your mind or that you are an "awful" person, or that people know your history or diagnosis because they can "just tell." As you pay attention, you may find other categories as well.

If someone has told you that you get paranoid but you aren't sure what the person means, ask the person or share your experience with your therapist so that, together, you can begin to get clearer about some of these thoughts.

■

Mindfulness Practice: Apply Nonjudgment and Stick to the Facts

When you are having thoughts of paranoia is an excellent time to practice sticking to the facts and being nonjudgmental. This works best if you can catch such thoughts early. When you notice your paranoid thoughts arising, begin your practice of labeling these thoughts *as* your paranoid thoughts. Find a quiet place and focus on your breath. If you notice intense emotions arising, you can use your grounding kit to feel more connected. Remember, paranoid thoughts are just thoughts, so be mindful not to judge yourself for having them. Ask yourself: *What are the facts of the situation? What evidence do I have?* Gently remind yourself that these are paranoid thoughts and you don't have to believe all of your thoughts. As you breathe, try to identify explanations or positions that are alternatives to the one that you are holding. If your thoughts go to concerns about your safety, remind yourself of where you are and what day, time, and year it is in order to, again, ground yourself in the facts of the reality in front of you.

While you are practicing this type of mindfulness, it can be helpful to make a list of your paranoid thoughts (when you are not experiencing them) and write down some nonjudgmental thoughts or ways to prompt your mind about how to work with them in the moment. After you have done this for a while, you may want to distract your mind with an activity, or use your grounding kit to help you remain present.

■

Mindfulness Practice: Notice and Label Thoughts, and Let Them Pass

Throughout the book you have been learning and practicing the following three skills: noticing thoughts, labeling them nonjudgmentally, and letting them pass without reacting. This exercise is similar to the previous one, only less active. You may begin to notice paranoid thoughts when you are out with friends or at work. This might be a challenging mindfulness practice, but it's one that you can try in the moment when you first notice the thoughts arise. The task of this practice is to notice when you are becoming paranoid, label your thought as "paranoid thought," and then let it pass, bringing your mind back to what you are doing. When the next thought arises, label it for what it is. You may use labels such as "paranoid thought," "worry thought," "future thought," and "past thought." This practice helps you to avoid getting caught up in the spiral of paranoid thinking and behaving. As you notice the intensity of the thoughts decrease, you may find that you gain mental clarity and have an easier time looking at the situation in front of you or returning to what you were doing without being as distracted.

■

Using mindfulness skills to work on your dissociation and paranoia can be challenging. Practicing your basic mindfulness skills will make applying them to these symptoms much easier. You may find that working with another person, such as your therapist, will help you to better understand how to identify symptoms of cognitive dysregulation and practice ways to use these mindfulness skills.

Chapter 9

Self-Dysregulation

Dysregulation of self includes the symptoms of identity disturbance, chronic feelings of emptiness, and self-hatred. This set of symptoms can be particularly hard to treat, because it's difficult to put precise words to such a deep and intense experience of who you are, especially an experience that causes such chronic misery. Using your mindfulness practice with these symptoms can be very challenging, because many people spend significant energy trying to avoid attending to these feelings, many hold judgments about themselves and this experience, and many have developed strong habits of avoidance to manage dysregulation of self.

If you want to end the symptoms associated with dysregulation of self, you need to have more than simply the desire to do so. You need to be willing. You have to be willing to see all of who you are: all of the parts, even those parts of yourself that you don't like. Many people with BPD refuse to acknowledge that there is anything redeeming about them or that they are kind, intelligent, or loyal. We are asking that you consider accepting all of who you are. Accept that the feelings you have about yourself are a part of you, and that you are open to them. Don't push them away. Until you can look at these feelings and see these parts of yourself, you cannot change them or view them differently. If you want change, you have to be willing to give your full attention. Freedom is living without fear and being able to face and ultimately accept the most painful parts of yourself. Emptiness and self-hatred are not you, but they are a part of you. Being willing to meet this process with love and compassion is your practice.

Identity Disturbance

Trying to figure out who we are is a developmental task normally found in adolescence and early adulthood. By age eighteen most people have begun to develop a cohesive and consistent sense of self. People with BPD do not always follow this typical developmental path and, as a result, experience a lack of knowing who they are. Amanda, a twenty-nine-year-old graduate student, described this:

> I know I'm a student, but I really I don't think I can answer the question of who I am or what kind of person I am. I am who is around me or what environment I am in, but I am never happy.
>
> I used to fight with my parents about buying too many clothes in high school and how many clubs I was in. My parents wanted me to settle down and find my place; they didn't understand that I never felt like I fit in. I tried being preppy. Then I hung out with the athletes, after which I joined the drama club. In tenth grade I was "emo" and wore all dark colors. Then I joined the gay-straight alliance, and the community service and environmental clubs. I needed environmentally friendly products, because I was a vegetarian and then a vegan. I never found my place.
>
> Now, as an adult, I do the same thing by getting different graduate degrees and jobs, and frequently coming up with different plans for my life.

The concept of identity can be quite confusing. When you have a sense of who you are, you know it, but when you don't, it can be hard to know what you are looking for. For years people have studied identity by using research and presenting theoretical models. A study on identity (Wilkinson-Ryan and Westen 2000) concluded that identity has the following elements and that they are underdeveloped in people with BPD:

- A stable sense of who you are, alone and in relationships

- A stable set of core values, morals, self-standards, and ideals

- The development of a worldview that provides you with an understanding of what gives life meaning

- Having others in your life who also recognize who you are and your place in the world

As we have discussed, people with BPD often lack consistency and report having different identities in different places and with different people.

"Who Am I?"

We have talked about the definition of identity on a broader level, which includes values, morals, ideals, and place in the world, but you also experience yourself on a more basic level through your thoughts, feelings, and body sensations. Those are your basic building blocks for getting to know who you are. Do you see the problem? People with BPD often have great difficulty with managing these building blocks and, in fact, spend more time avoiding, judging, and suppressing these building blocks than using them.

Applying Mindfulness Skills for Identity Disturbance

Many people with BPD have told us that they just don't feel comfortable in their own skin. That is, they do not feel that they can genuinely experience themselves without reacting in some way, often to fears or perceived needs in the moment. Mindfulness will help you go back to the building blocks and develop your ability to not only begin to feel more comfortable in your own skin, but also get to know what's inside your skin so that you can begin to pay attention to what matters and what's important to you, and learn how to live accordingly.

Mindfulness Practice: Notice and Label How You Change

As we have discussed, people with BPD often feel as if they take on different roles with changing goals and values, without awareness in the moment. As you now know, mindfulness starts with awareness, so we would like for you to pay attention and notice how you change. Set aside some time and make a list of ways that you change. Do this task with curiosity and nonjudgment, again as if you were a researcher collecting data. Once you have made your list, commit to paying attention to how you change for one week, and add your observations to the list. This practice will help you start to become aware of patterns, which, as you have heard before, is the first step. As you build awareness, you can begin to notice changes in the moment, and pause to evaluate how to proceed. You will learn ways to evaluate your next steps in later practices.

- *Do you frequently change your goals? Have you set goals, started to complete the steps to achieve those goals, and then given up and changed to something else? Does this happen over and over again? Are your goals affected by what other people think or how you feel in the moment? What are some of the things that make you change your goals?*

- *Do you have changing values and behaviors? Think about times when you may have committed to something or acted in a way that surprised you or made you feel uncomfortable or guilty afterward. Do you act differently with different people?*

- *Do you take on different identities in different situations? Do you dress or speak differently? How would different people in your life describe you?*

■

Mindfulness Practice: Learn What's Important to You

What's important to you? It's not uncommon for this question to evoke anxiety and a quick "I don't know" response. We are asking you to use your notice-and-label skills when emotions such as anxiety, fear, and sadness arise, and, instead of reacting or avoiding, to stay present in the moment as you work on this practice. Figuring out what's important to you is a process, and for some, just the thought of it can be so overwhelming that they give up. Knowing what is important to you will give you a foundation to evaluate your behaviors moving forward, instead of using other people as an ever-changing foundation.

Relying on other people's values when they don't fit your own can cause a lot of suffering and, at times, lead to self-destructive and dangerous behaviors. This means that as you think about what's important to you, you will need to notice whether thoughts about other people's reactions arise, as well as notice the patterns you have become aware of from the previous practice. Again, use your noticing skills and label these thoughts "What other people will think thoughts." Then come back to what's important to you. You will also need to use your "doing one thing in the moment" skill, because your mind may wander quickly to how you will achieve these goals. Remember, the intention of this task is to make a list of what's important to you, because you need that before you can make a plan. Pay attention to what this process is like.

Spend some time in a quiet place that you find comfortable, and sit in a mindful, grounded position. Using a journal or notebook, begin by answering the following questions:

1. *How do I want to treat people in my life?*

2. *What impact do I want to have on others?*

3. *What are my views on politics, religion, education, and family?*

4. *How do I think about these things?*

5. *What kind of school or work do I want to pursue?*

6. *How do I want others to see me?*

7. *What contributions do I want to make?*

As you work on this practice, you may find more questions that you would like to answer. Remember, you can repeat this practice a couple of times and add to it. The practice is essentially both building a list, and staying present and curious about what's important to you at times when you alone.

■

Mindfulness Practice: Find Your Breath

Breath work is a foundation practice of mindfulness, and it's your most powerful tool for helping yourself to stay grounded and remain in your own skin. The beauty of your breath is that it's always with you and you can always bring your attention back to it. You can find yourself with your breath. Remember that paying attention to your breath is a way to slow down your thinking and your reactions so that you can connect with yourself and what's important to you.

Find a quiet place and sit in your mindful position. This practice is about counting your breaths. Some people use only numbers; others prefer to count using an image, such as climbing up a set of stairs or a ladder. Beginning with a two-minute practice, you will count your inhalation and exhalation as one, then your next set of breaths as two, and so on.

Try to follow your breathing instead of making your breathing fit your counting. This means that your inhalations and exhalations may be uneven. Don't worry if your breathing starts to match your counting; as you continue to practice, this will get easier. For this practice, you will count to ten. When your mind wanders, which it will, or you find yourself counting beyond ten, start at one again. Each time you notice your mind getting distracted, bring your attention back to the task of counting and begin at one. For some people, when you catch your mind in distraction, it can be useful to say to yourself, *Wandering mind,* and then return to inhaling and counting from one.

The goal for this practice is not necessarily to reach ten, but to notice your mind wander, catch it, and bring it back. The act of bringing your mind back, not simply having a quiet mind, is mindfulness. You will need your skills of nonjudgment here as well. Remember, your mind produces thoughts, so it will continue to do so. When we do this practice, it's not often that either of us reaches ten.

You may be asking what this has to do with identity. This practice helps you to stay in your skin and in your experience without reacting. This practice can also help you to get connected to your intuition or what is called your "wise mind" in DBT (Linehan 1993). Your intuition helps you to connect to your values, morals, needs, and wants. We recommend doing this as a daily practice and seeing if over time, you can increase the duration of this practice, adding thirty seconds or a minute each week.

Once you begin to do this practice formally, you can use it in your daily life to help slow down your reactions. For example, before agreeing to do something, making a big change in your life, or having an emotionally charged conversation, find your breath, slow yourself down, breathe, stay in the present moment, and then assess your own thoughts and feelings before taking action. This gives you time to assess whether your behavior fits with your own goals and values so that you avoid reacting to thoughts and emotions. The goal is to build your own sense of who you are and stay steady, even when you notice urges to sacrifice your own identity for someone else's. Because this is a new behavior, you may notice that other people begin to react to and treat you differently as well.

■

Chronic Feelings of Emptiness

When Ann, a twenty-three-year-old college senior, came to the clinic seeking help for her BPD, the aspect she struggled most with was how empty she felt:

I feel so empty inside. I try to fill the emptiness with people and activities, but it only lasts a while and then I feel empty again. Cocaine, sex, and online gaming seem to help for a while, but they are distractions. I can't find a nice, stable guy; I have to find guys whose lives are full of drama. That excites me for a while, but I know it's not healthy. I know it; I just can't stop myself.

If not with lovers, drugs, or other distractions, how do you deal with emptiness? Of all of the *DSM* criteria for diagnosing BPD, perhaps the most difficult symptom to explain to others is having chronic feelings of emptiness. Emptiness is such a subjective experience, and people with BPD know it when they feel it. Other symptoms, such as anger, black-and-white thinking, and impulsivity are easier for others to see, but trying to explain your sense of emptiness to someone who has never experienced it can seem nearly impossible. The criterion of emptiness is present in more than 70 percent of people with BPD (Grilo et al. 2001). Research shows that feelings of emptiness often precede suicide attempts (Schnyder et al. 1999), and yet this criterion has not been well studied.

What Is Emptiness?

Asking someone with BPD to describe the feeling of emptiness draws many responses. Some describe an unbearable void: a hopelessness and purposelessness that leads them to the conclusion that they are of no consequence and that the world would be better off without them. For others, emptiness feels like a part of who they are. Others experience it as philosophical or existential. A twenty-five-year-old grad student described it this way:

For me it's a lack of meaning, a lack of purpose, and a lack of motivation. I feel so numb that it hurts. It really sucks. It's a giant hole. It feels as if nothing I do could fill it. I used to think emptiness was because people didn't understand me, but even when I met other people with BPD, I still felt the hole in my life. I look for other things to fill it, but even when I get what I want, it lasts for a few days and I need more. Nothing ever seems to be enough. But here is where it gets worse: even when I'm busy, I feel like I'm only distracting myself from the hole in my life. So what can I do?

For others, emptiness is a very specific experience, like feeling completely alone despite being in a group of people or crying in the belief that nothing is ever going to change. For many, there's no escape. Moving from one situation to the next or from one environment to another simply brings the feeling with you. A nineteen-year-old explained:

Emptiness is like my skin. It goes with me everywhere. Here's what it is. It's not knowing who I am or what I feel or need. It's feeling that I don't mean anything to anyone, that I have nothing to contribute to society or to relationships. What's the point in having a goal if it doesn't mean anything? But without a goal, there's no future. It goes around and around. I feel empty, so nothing means anything, so I don't have a goal, so I don't have a future, so my life is empty. Crazy, right? But that's how it feels.

I used to cut. That brought me back to reality, because then I had a goal of not cutting! Being alone is also part of it. When I am completely close to someone, it helps a bit, but no one can stay glued to you, and when the person leaves, the abandonment kicks in. Emptiness is a horrible way to live, and there's very little relief from it.

So what does emptiness mean to you? Is it loneliness or a feeling of not fitting in? When you pay attention to the experience of emptiness, what thoughts and feelings come up for you?

Emptiness in BPD

If you find it difficult to explain emptiness, you are not alone; researchers on the subject have a similar problem. This is because emptiness can be difficult to define and assess. In therapy, your therapist might try to get at it by using examples from others who suffer from BPD. Words are often imprecise approximations of what you actually feel. In 2008 psychologist David Klonsky studied the nature of emptiness. He and his colleagues were able to more clearly define aspects of emptiness in the context of BPD, and found that:

- Emptiness is closely related to feelings of hopelessness, loneliness, and isolation.

- There's a big overlap between emptiness and hopelessness. Hopelessness is a strong risk factor for suicide, so emptiness puts people with BPD at risk for suicide.

- Emptiness is more strongly related to suicidal thinking than any other BPD criterion. It appears that chronic emptiness contributes to the development of suicidal thoughts, although emptiness itself does not appear to move suicidal thoughts to suicide attempts.

- Emptiness and boredom are not the same thing. This is an important finding, because therapists often imagine that they are, and often use the ideas interchangeably.

- Chronic emptiness seems to overlap a great deal with depression but not with anxiety.

Temporary Relief

For many people who feel empty, the easiest and quickest relief is to act reactively and to do something that distracts from the intolerable feeling. Impulsive and self-destructive behaviors such as self-injury, substance use, and sex can act as short distractions from this intense feeling. It may seem unfair that you experience such feelings more than other people do, and you may be able to use mindfulness to help.

We have talked a lot about the problems with behaving reactively, without awareness. Some ways of distracting are healthier, and people tell us that keeping busy with work or school helps. For others, the distractions are less healthy. Some get involved in quick, intense relationships, hoping that the relationship will end the feeling. As with many quick solutions, a new relationship can temporarily relieve emptiness, but people with BPD find that this doesn't tend to last. Even when you stay in a new relationship, the emptiness can creep back in and haunt you.

Stephanie, a thirty-two-year-old mother of two daughters, said:

When it gets too intense, that's when I feel my most borderline. I have to get away from the feeling, because in the past, it led me to suicidal thinking. It [suicide] was an option before I had the girls, but I would never do that to them. What I do is go to work. On weekends I clean the house, watch TV, do crosswords, and try to go to the gym. Sometimes I call my mother, and sometimes that helps, but other times I end up feeling more lonely and misunderstood.

Applying Mindfulness Skills to Chronic Emptiness

So, where do you begin to apply your mindfulness skills to feelings of emptiness? Your first practice is to get to know your emptiness. Notice whether right about now, feelings of skepticism are rising as we direct you to pay attention to such a painful feeling. If so, that makes sense, and we ask you to notice your reaction and perhaps your fear, and open your mind to the following task. Most of us get to know other people or information by asking questions. See if you can step back as an observer and think about your experiences of emptiness. Here are some questions to ask yourself about emptiness: *How does the feeling of emptiness prevent me from living the life I want to live? What are my judgments about emptiness? What is my goal in addressing emptiness?*

Mindfulness Practice: Pay Attention to Your Emptiness

You have learned a number of different ways to pay attention. Here's an opportunity to practice intentionally noticing and labeling your experience of emptiness. This is a challenging practice, because for many people with BPD, the feelings associated with emptiness are judged as not only bad, but also constant. We are asking you to essentially stare down your "enemy."

Paying attention to emptiness is easiest when there's not much to distract you. You may be surprised at what thoughts and feelings emerge when you pay attention to emptiness. As you are learning this practice, it's best to find a quiet place, somewhere in your house or outside. As with other practices, begin by doing this one when you are experiencing emptiness that's not so intense. Many people with BPD describe a low-level, or chronic, aching around emptiness as well as some discrete times of increased intensity. If that's the case for you, begin by drawing your attention to emptiness at the lower, or aching, level so that you don't find yourself overcome by the intensity of emptiness before you become better skilled at mindfulness practice.

As you become more skilled at this practice and less judgmental about emptiness, you will be able to practice this skill in the moment and at times when your emptiness is most intense. This practice will help you avoid responding to your emptiness with short-term or self-destructive solutions.

Find a quiet place and begin by focusing on your breath. Slowly bring your awareness to the feeling of emptiness. Notice that you are deliberately focusing and not avoiding, and see what thoughts and judgments arise. You will begin to see that this experience is made up of many thoughts and emotions, and that if you can let them, they will change.

Your practice will be to notice and label the thoughts and emotions. When you experience a thought like *I feel empty,* say to yourself, *Thought about emptiness.* When you notice a judgmental thought like *This is so bad,* say to yourself, *Judgmental thought.* When you have thoughts about the future or the past, such as *I will always be alone* or *No one has ever understood me,* label them *Thought about the future* and *Thought about the past.* You will do the same thing with emotions. When you notice a feeling arise, label it as such—for example, *feeling of sadness.* Labeling gives you the ability to pause and prevent your thoughts from spiraling out of control. It is a small but powerful act.

You may find this practice tedious, and it will help you to slow down and attend to the whole experience so that you can get more information and better understand your emptiness. Notice that your mind has all of these thoughts, that they merely exist in your head, and that they come and go. You may also begin to experience an increase in the intensity of the thoughts and feelings. Some people find that the intensity increases like a wave, and if you can ride the wave until it peaks, then you find that, like a wave, the intensity decreases as it crashes on the shore. Here's the magic. Simply observing all of this will allow you to realize that thoughts and feelings around emptiness change, which is an important fact that's often forgotten.

This practice will allow you to realize that although the thought that you are empty may not feel pleasant the thought doesn't *make* you empty. You will realize that you and "empty" are not the same thing. Remember, our brains often convince us that we are our thoughts and feelings, and then we hold on and become attached to that meaning. When you can "get" this practice, you will find tremendous freedom and an increased ability to let thoughts and feelings simply be thoughts and feelings that come and go.

■

Mindfulness Practice: Accept Reality As It Is

As we discussed before, accepting reality as it is—what Marsha Linehan calls "radical acceptance" (Linehan 1993)—can be one of the hardest mindfulness skills to practice. Nonacceptance is often at the root of our suffering and at the root of all BPD symptoms. We have found that feelings of emptiness are some of the most harshly judged and least accepted by people with BPD. What's curious is that one of the most uncomfortable and challenging symptoms for BPD sufferers is one that they inadvertently make worse through nonacceptance. You will remember that practicing acceptance doesn't mean agreeing with or liking something; it means accepting what is in this moment. Practicing acceptance can profoundly influence our own behavior and can decrease distress. When you work on accepting something, you can begin to step back and see the bigger picture, learn about your role in the situation, and see patterns of behavior. When you move toward acceptance, you begin to feel less trapped in your experience, which allows you to deal with reality as it is and then let it change.

Many people have strong reactions and nonacceptance around feelings of emptiness, because emptiness feels intolerable. That nonacceptance and its accompanying judgments only enhance and prolong your feelings. For most people, the reaction to feeling empty is immediate nonacceptance and urges to take action to rid themselves of the feeling by engaging in some sort of distraction. Remember, distraction is avoidance, and it will only provide you with a short-term solution. At times, you may choose a short-term solution; what's important is that making that choice is done with awareness and isn't simply an automatic reaction.

This is an exercise for you to practice when you find yourself in a place of nonacceptance. Before you do this practice, it's important that you know when you are fighting reality. Thoughts such as *I shouldn't feel like this, I shouldn't have to deal with this, It's not fair,* and *If only _____, then I wouldn't feel like this,* and judgments such as *I hate this, This will never end,* and *I can't stand this* are all signals to yourself that you are not accepting reality as it is. This exercise is a useful way to help you work toward acceptance when you are feeling empty, and with that acceptance, you will find change.

As with most of our exercises, we encourage you to practice this exercise in times of lower emotional intensity, around something that you are having a hard time accepting or simply when you think about the symptom of emptiness. The goal is for you to be able to use this practice in moments of intense feelings of emptiness that might be emphasized by your lack of acceptance. As with all mindfulness exercises, the more you practice, the stronger the effect can be and the more accessible the practice will be in times of distress.

Set a timer to beep at two-minute intervals. Sit in a quiet place in a mindful, grounded, and open position. For eight minutes you are going to think of *emptiness.* As you become more practiced, you can do this in your day-to-day life, when your feelings of emptiness become intense and may be inter-fering with your day.

In your mind, repeat, *I don't like it*. After two minutes or so, repeat, *I can't change it* for two more minutes. Then say, *I can accept it*. For the last two minutes, say, *I will accept it*.

■

Mindfulness Practice: Connect with Others

When you feel empty, alone, and disconnected, you might be falling into a mental trap. Now this may seem a bit abstract, but fundamentally we are all interconnected and dependent on each other. For some people who struggle with strong urges to carry out self-destructive behaviors or suicide, this idea can be another set of thoughts that you avoid. Paying attention to your connection with others can be challenging for a couple of reasons: First, when you are feeling emptiest, it can be difficult to consider the connections that you have in your life because you experience them as absent. Second, paying attention to connectedness means paying attention to the impact that you have on others and how many people you and your behaviors can affect in a positive and a negative way. You rely on others, and others rely on you, even when it isn't all that obvious. Your connection and impact cascade, and unless you pay attention to them, they are easy to miss. Feelings of emptiness often shut off the capacity to attend to your connectedness. Your mindfulness practice is to turn this ability back on. To do this, you must practice paying attention to your connectedness.

1. Think about the people who rely on you—for example, your local coffee-shop employees, who depend in part on your business; your spouse or

partner, who has expectations; your employer, who depends on your being at work every day; your teacher, who needs a class full of students in order to teach.

2. Spend a few minutes making a list of your connections, and see how far you can reach out in identifying them. Challenge your mind to begin thinking this way.

In Buddhist philosophy the act and skill of realizing that you are not isolated, but instead are intimately connected to everything, is fundamental. Building your capacity to observe your connectedness will help liberate you from the trap of believing what your mind has created, including the trap of emptiness.

■

Self-Hatred

Pervasive feelings of self-hatred are all too common in people with BPD. We frequently hear that someone feels that she is simply the worst and stupidest person in the world. Maya, a twenty-seven-year-old with BPD, said the following:

You don't understand; I'm awful and destructive. I ruin people's lives; there's no one who's as horrible as I am. No one would love someone like me, and you cannot possibly care about someone as ugly and disgusting as I am. If you understood, you wouldn't come near me. You probably don't and couldn't care about me anyway. I am probably just a pity case, because you see that I am so awful.

This is felt with such intensity that people have lowered themselves to holding the spot of the worst or most-hated person in the world.

While there are many problems with self-hatred, one of the biggest ones is that it unilaterally increases a person's suffering. You may also notice that feelings of self-hatred color the way you experience or view negative events in your life, such as pain or failure. While not directly addressed in DBT, practicing compassion is an integral part of the Buddhist mindfulness practice and one of the paths to freedom from suffering. Perhaps you are finding this concept to be quite foreign. From a mindfulness perspective, self-hatred is also a practice and one that you may be quite skilled at, even if it's causing you misery.

Research has shown that for adolescents and adults, self-compassion is correlated with increased well-being, social connectedness, and life satisfaction; and decreased depression, anxiety, self-criticism, rumination, and thought suppression (Barnard and Curry 2011). Moreover, research shows that self-compassion eases the impact of negative events in our lives. It sounds pretty important, doesn't it? When you can take a self-compassionate position during times of failure, you are more likely to be able to see your role or shortcomings and, instead of obsessing, overidentifying, and self-criticizing, view this as a time for sympathy and support, and even an opportunity to do something differently next time. People who are more self-compassionate are less afraid of failure (Germer 2009).

Self-Compassion

When you experience pain, disappointment, or failure, your mind produces many different types of thoughts and feelings about yourself. Self-compassion is a practice for these difficult times, and it has three components (Neff 2003):

- Being kind and understanding toward yourself when you are in pain or experience failure, rather than being self-critical

- Seeing that everyone is fallible and that fallibility is part of the human condition rather than an isolating experience

- Holding painful thoughts and feelings in mindful awareness, rather than avoiding, suppressing, or overidentifying with these thoughts and feelings

Some people have already learned the practice of self-compassion, so it comes more easily, but for many people with BPD, this practice is a particular challenge. When you pay attention, you will see that your response to yourself when you are in pain has a powerful impact on how much you suffer. Thus, those who struggle and are in pain often need self-compassion the most, and happen to be the people least likely to use it. Self-hatred is an obstacle to finding self-compassion and, thus, prolongs suffering. It's a vicious cycle.

While the concept of self-compassion may be new, the components likely sound familiar (nonjudgment, expanding your awareness to see the larger picture, and noticing and labeling nonreactively), so your previous knowledge of mindfulness will help with this practice. Like all mindfulness skills, self-compassion is developed gradually through practice, so it's important to pay attention to the gradual changes that occur.

Applying Mindfulness Skills to Self-Hatred

Self-hatred is a powerful experience filled with self-judgment. The mindfulness skills for self-hatred are equally powerful and therefore can be exceptionally challenging to practice. These skills will challenge you to practice a way of treating yourself that may feel antithetical to your nature. However, you will learn much more about yourself when you take a more mindful and curious stance, and do so with kindness and compassion.

Meeting Self-Hatred with Kindness

In chapter 4, we introduced Sharon Salzberg, a leading spiritual teacher and author who is credited for bringing the ancient Buddhist practice of metta, or loving-kindness meditation, to the West. She believes that kindness is compassion in action. The art of practicing kindness means being able to evoke feelings of empathy and sympathy within yourself in the most difficult situation that you witness and experience, with the goal of decreasing your own suffering (Salzberg 2010). Imagine bringing self-kindness to feelings of loneliness, emptiness, abandonment, or disappointment.

Some people have judgments about kindness and regard it as resignation, agreement, or weakness. This is not the practice we are talking about. This practice asks you to find power in kindness, control over your own experience, and the ability to stick to your values in the face of difficulties. Being able to do this increases your ability to help others. So, how do you do it? The following practices will focus on building your capacity to be kind to yourself. In contrast to judgment and criticism, you will be building feelings of empathy, gentleness, warmth, forgiveness, and patience with yourself and others when you confront suffering.

Mindfulness Practice: Metta (Loving-Kindness)

The practice of metta is done by reciting a series of meaningful phrases about treating yourself and others with kindness. The metta practice typically consists of repeating four phrases that have the following themes: freedom from danger, mental happiness, physical happiness, and ease of living and wellbeing. Sharon Salzberg provides the following template (Salzberg 2008, 37):

- *May I be free from danger.*

- *May I have mental happiness.*

- *May I have physical happiness.*

- *May I have ease of well-being.*

The idea is to experiment with these phrases and make them your own. We will share one of ours and encourage you to change the phrases in a way that feels meaningful and useful to you. You will first practice directing your metta practice toward yourself, and then you can extend the practice to others.

In your practice, you may use the previous phrases or the following ones, which are our modifications:

- *May I be filled with loving-kindness.*

- *May I be free.*

- *May I be peaceful and at ease.*

- *May I be happy.*

Before you begin, write out your metta phrases and bring them to your practice. Find a quiet place and sit mindfully. Set your timer for three minutes. Begin by taking a few mindful breaths, and set your intention to let feelings of kindness arise, noticing the good within yourself. After taking a few breaths, begin to recite your phrases to yourself. Use a gentle tone and a comfortable pace, remembering that you are offering kindness to yourself. You can coordinate the phrases with your breath if that's helpful, but it's not required. In the beginning, you may simply read the phrases you've written. You will find that in time, you can recite them from memory. When you find that your mind has become distracted from your practice, gently bring it back and begin reciting from the beginning. When you finish your practice, pay attention, noticing and labeling your experience.

Once you have sufficient practice at offering loving-kindness to yourself, you can extend your practice to others, such as a loved one who has supported you; a neutral person in your life—for example, the person who made your coffee or bagged your groceries; someone in your life who is suffering; someone whom you are having a difficult time with; and then all beings. When you practice metta, you will always begin by offering loving-kindness to yourself and then to others. So, you may set your timer for three minutes and offer loving-kindness to yourself, and then use the next three minutes to offer it to someone else, and so on. Remember, when you offer your phrase to others, visualize the person and replace the "I" in your phrase with that person's name or image. In other words, if you have a friend named John, replace the "I" in your phrase with the word "John," or replace the word "I" with an image of John. This is a powerful practice, which we hope you will return to often.

■

Mindfulness Practice: Acts of Kindness toward Yourself

We have talked about how behavior can be a powerful mechanism for change. For this practice we ask that for one week, you make a commitment to doing something kind for yourself each day. These don't need to be large acts, but rather small gestures like treating yourself to a cup of coffee, taking a bath, making time to attend a yoga or exercise class that you enjoy, cooking yourself your favorite meal, buying yourself some fresh flowers, or opening that candle or bottle of wine that you had been saving for something special. Make some space to be gentle with yourself, and pay attention to your mood and thoughts after each act.

■

Mindfulness Practice: Random Acts of Kindness

Self-hatred often comes with powerful stories and feelings of worthlessness, uselessness, and meaninglessness. You stop noticing the positive impact that you have on others and what it feels like to make a contribution to others. This is a powerful reminder of the transactional impact of kindness. Set your intention to practice a certain number of random acts of kindness each week. The powerful part of this practice is that your acts are random, without expectation of anything in return. The most effective acts can be with people you don't know. If you are having difficulty identifying random acts, consider things like helping someone carry groceries, secretly paying for both your coffee and that of the person behind you in line, putting money in an expired meter, or simply smiling and saying hello to someone you walk past. Again, notice your experience after each of these acts.

■

Common Humanity vs. Isolation

Earlier we discussed how one aspect of self-compassion is being able to step back and see that failure is part of the human condition. Interestingly, in DBT all therapists agree on a number of fundamental assumptions, one of which is that all therapists are fallible and therefore will make mistakes and disappoint people (Linehan 1993). So, we will challenge you to make this assumption as well. People with BPD often struggle with perfectionism and overidentify with failures, disappointments, and inadequacies. They have difficulty seeing that, in fact, imperfection and failure are fundamental parts of being human. It is our responses to failures and mistakes, however, that dictate our suffering much of the time. Feeling isolated, alone, or unique in your failures is extremely painful and simply not true. This can be a very tricky practice, because the goal is not to invalidate your experience or compare it to those who suffer worse, but to step back and remind yourself that your feelings of inadequacy are valid *and* shared. When you can step back and see that you are not alone in these experiences, you can look at yourself with more kindness, which can help you to find others who are similar to you so that you don't feel as isolated. This is an act of accepting that you, too, are human.

Mindfulness Practice: Common Humanity

Take some time to think about something that you consider to be a small failure. Recall the experience and what it felt like. Now, as you breathe, notice the feelings and sensations in your body. Remind yourself of the following things: *While some people may appear to have it easier then I do, no one can avoid failure. I know that failure and imperfection are a painful part of being human. There are people out there who share my feelings, and I am not alone; I am simply human, like everyone else.* The goal is to practice enough for these feelings to expand into your daily life so that you can begin to tackle failures and disappointments in the moment in a way that decreases your suffering and self-hatred.

■

You have learned different ways to practice mindfulness to address the many symptoms of BPD, and it is our hope that you will return to these practices over and over again. The final part of this book will look ahead to the journey you are beginning as you embark on the mindfulness path.

Part 4

The Journey Ahead

Chapter 10

Telling the Story of Your Life

Most of us are introduced to stories at a very young age. Parents, grandparents, older siblings, babysitters, and teachers read us stories until we learn to read for ourselves. Stories are based on reality or fiction, and can teach, instruct, or simply entertain and hold a reader's interest.

As we get older, we begin to tell ourselves our own stories, and among other things, these stories can serve to calm us down, justify our behavior, validate our experiences, provide encouragement, protect us from something we fear, or make the uncertain certain. Some of these stories are useful, and others lead to enduring suffering. Telling these stories without awareness can be quite dangerous, and many people forget that at some level, these stories are fiction, often a narrow and judgmental account of the past or predictions about the future. Many people with BPD tell such stories as if the stories were accurate representations, and they do so without awareness, getting swept away by powerful thoughts and feelings. A particular challenge is that people with BPD often feel a strong attachment to their stories, even those that bring them tremendous misery.

Part of the mindfulness path is to pay attention to your stories in a way that helps you determine whether it's effective. When you begin to pay attention, you will learn that, in fact, you are both the author and the editor of your story, and you have the power to change it. In this final chapter you will put your mindfulness skills to work as you look at your stories and how they influence how you view your past, live in the present, and predict your future.

BPD Stories

Often when we introduce the idea of storytelling in therapy, we get a fair amount of "pushback." It's as if we were threatening to take away something sacred. It can feel like this when you are very attached to your stories and your ways of explaining your life and reactions. Remember, the power of the stories you tell yourself is in how they influence not only your emotions, but also your behavior. Stories about the future, as bleak as they may be, can alleviate anxiety about the unknown, even though they cause misery. For some, a story of absolute failure may feel more tolerable than the fear of trying and failing. For many people with BPD, that misery and suffering are familiar, which can feel safer than the uncertainty of the unknown. Often it's your stories and how you tell them that keep you stuck.

"My Life: This Is How It Always Goes"

We all have our stories, and people with BPD often find themselves telling similar stories to account for symptoms and ongoing suffering. The following are a few examples.

Sydney, who is thirty-two and has been diagnosed with BPD, was living with the following story. This story would show up whenever Sydney started, ended, or was involved in a relationship. It went something like this:

Who could ever love me? I know my parents didn't love me.
I was unlovable then; I should have known. No one can really
love someone like me. I am meant to be alone, and really,
I deserve it. I mess up relationships and other people. When
things are going well, it's because they don't really know me.
I know that sooner or later, everyone will realize what a terrible

*person I am, and then they will just leave me. I will always
be alone, so what's the point?*

Amber is a twenty-year-old who was diagnosed with BPD. She
was declined admission to college and has developed the following
story, which has kept her from repeating the application process. Her
story goes like this:

*No colleges want me. I am stupid and can't do it anyway.
Teachers have always hated me, because I'm just not smart.
When I get good grades, it's just because they pity me because
I have problems; they want to get rid of me, so they pass me.
I know there are a lot of colleges, but even if I did get in somewhere, I would just fail because that's what happens to people
like me. I'll never be good enough for my family, so what's the
point anyway? I just can't do it, and I don't see why people want
me to try.*

Mara is a twenty-seven-year-old with a powerful story that plagues
her in times of loneliness and self-loathing:

*I am so desperate. I'm a worthless person, and I am not even sure
why people even bother with me. How can you help me if I am
the worst person who ever lived? What a bleak life I live. I am so
alone. I am alone even when I am with my friends, and when
I'm not with them, I am lonely and no one understands that.
Worse is that no one wants me, because who would want such
a miserable person? People hate me. I am so toxic to the world
I poison it, but people won't tell that to someone's face. I am
repulsive and attention seeking, which is why I have hurt so
many people. I am destructive. I know people hate me, and
I wonder why people don't bother to tell me. Everybody would
be better off if I was dead. No one would care, and people close
to me will get over it; they are stronger than I am. Change won't
help, because if you are the worst person in the world, that's your
lot in life and you remain that even if you change some. I hate
myself; I am useless.*

Like the rest of us, Sydney, Amber, and Mara become the stories they tell themselves. Such stories become ingrained, define you, and influence your behaviors. Stories lock you into a certain identity. Further, the more you tell yourself the story, the more you believe it and the better you get at telling it. Eventually it becomes hardwired into your sense of who you are. Every one of us has a story to tell, but the story can be told in many ways. Stories are the way in which you connect the *you* that you recount and the people in your world. The types of stories that people with BPD tell themselves develop in the depth of their misery or late at night in a tired mind. But then the stories are perpetuated.

How do you tell your story? What aspects do you focus on? What you tell yourself and others is a choice. Do you tend to focus only on the negative, recounting a past filled with pain and failure? Are there no happy memories or stories? Are the endings always the same?

Life Is Not a Static Tale

Any one of us can be convinced that there is some absolute truth about our lives. You might be certain that absolutes exist. Do you tell yourself stories that are unchanging, that repeat the same script over and over again, and do you believe that it's the only way to tell your story?

Often we see politicians and the clergy insisting that there's only one way. So many people claim to know the way, and all too often, these ways are contradicting. This is inevitable because we live in a world with multiple cultures, multiple religions, and multiple individuals. Time, space, and resources change how we think, so even though there are rules about marriage, evolution, abortion, teen pregnancy, drugs, and so on, every one of these mores will change because society changes. For instance, here are rules that, at one point, our society was certain about:

Women voting: Before 1920 women did not have the right to vote in the United States, and in many other countries today, women still do not have that right.

Racial segregation: This has been a "fact" of life and law throughout history, and there are still groups that believe that there should be segregation.

Slavery: For thousands of years, our religious books have told stories of slaves, and in the past, laws protected the right to own slaves in the United States.

Polygamy: Many countries, religions, and cultures practice polygamy, but in many other countries, it's illegal.

And just as society changes, so will your brain. With new information, you change, and the only way to perpetuate stories is to keep telling them without opening your mind to the possibility that there are other ways to explain what happened, and other alternatives for how you can feel or think about your life and your future.

As for all of us, your interpretation of the world that you live in, and your sense of identity, is rooted in the story you have told, and because you don't pay attention to the telling, you believe the story to be factual. The problem is that the story often leaves you miserable and stuck.

Applying Mindfulness Skills to Telling Your Story

Awareness and the telling of your story will challenge you to use all of your mindfulness skills. You must choose to attentively look at your stories and do so without judgment. You will be challenged to notice and label without judgment, to stay grounded in the present, and to take a one-mindful, one-thing-in-the-moment, approach. This is not a small challenge but one to approach with curiosity and openness.

Mindfulness Practice: How You Choose to Tell It—EDIT

In order to change your story, become an editor. Use the acronym EDIT to look at some of your stories. What do you notice when you edit the story and change the outcome? Practice being nonjudgmental and compassionate.

1. Express your story on paper, mindfully attending to habitual details.

2. Describe the ways in which specific assumptions lead to specific thoughts and emotions.

3. Identify the thoughts and emotions that cause you the most suffering.

4. Tell your story differently, use different assumptions, and end the story differently.

Pay attention to when your story shows up; notice it and label it as simply a story, one that you have repeated many times about events that have not yet happened; and bring your mind back to the present.

■

Mindfulness Practice: No Need to Suffer Twice

Imagine that you have a job interview in a few hours. The interview exists in the future. You might tell yourself the story that you are going to fail the interview and never get the job. There are a few possibilities. One is that you do well and get the job. In this scenario, you suffer needlessly from telling yourself that story. Another possibility is that you don't get the job and then suffer from the disappointment. In this scenario you suffer twice, once from worrying about the outcome and then, again, from the actual outcome. If you are going to suffer, there's no need to suffer twice. Do you find yourself suffering when there's no need to?

■

Mindfulness Practice: How You Choose to Tell It—Find Alternatives

Imagine being at an uncreative job that you don't like and your friends encouraging you to switch to a job that requires artistic talent. Everyone, except for you, recognizes that you are gifted, so the story begins. You tell your friends:

I'll never make it. I suck at art. In any case, even if I somehow got an interview, they would never hire me because my résumé is lousy. I tried switching jobs before and failed. You guys just don't get it! I should just stick it out in my crappy job.

In these statements you are predicting the future. How could you tell this story differently? In this practice, notice and label the statements that you make and the way in which you tell your story. If you are having a hard time remembering the things that you tend to say, ask your friends. Now take each statement and retell it in a less absolute and more factual way.

Statement	Alternative Statement
■ *I'll never make it.*	_____
■ *I suck at art.*	_____
■ *They will never hire me.*	_____
■ *My résumé is lousy.*	_____
■ *You guys don't get it.*	_____

Are your original statements "the truth"? It's easy to get caught up in the belief that past experiences will predict the future, but many of these statements aren't factual; they are judgments. Take a nonjudgmental stance. If you want to learn, you need to perceive your situation without judgment.

The other problem is that if you have come to the conclusion that you are going to fail anyway, then you lose the opportunity to try to find a way to succeed. And then the more you tell yourself you are going to fail, the more you are practicing the story and the more you will believe it. In fact, the only way to make certain that you fail is to not attempt the task at all. You have to stop telling yourself all the reasons you are going to fail, or at least notice these thoughts and recognize that they are often judgment-filled conclusions.

■

Choosing How You Experience Your Life

After a year of DBT and focusing on mindfulness, Devon, who has experienced a life of self-deprecation and self-doubt, reflects on the recovery process:

> I used to think in terms of good and bad, but now I recognize good and bad as judgments. Today I still get caught up that way, but not so often. I use mindfulness to recognize the judgment, and now I think in terms of what's effective and ineffective— what actually works for me! Thinking in this way means that the negative stories that I have repeated, the ones that say You are a failure, and you'll never do anything right, are no longer prominent. So even though my journey has not been an easy one, I have gotten to a place of accepting my life. My experience is different now. I don't suffer as much, even when there is suffering, and believe me, there is still suffering. I now know who I am,

I know what my values are, and, these days, I like myself more.
I feel loved by my friends, I feel deserving of that love,
and I have let go of having to know what will happen.

The Mindful Journey

Your journey through life with BPD is not a life that is destined to be one of suffering and misery, even though at times you may feel that it is. Not every one of the practices in the book will help, and some may seem impossible, but in reading this book, you have taken your first steps along the mindfulness path. The journey ahead of you is one where you will begin to practice living with your eyes wide open to the present moment as it unfolds before you. You can begin to notice patterns and to do things differently, approaching outcomes with curiosity and compassion. At times, this practice will test long-standing beliefs about yourself and the world around you. This is a challenging journey on a winding path. You will use your awareness to notice when you have let go of the practice, and gently come back to your breath and the skills you have learned. The best advice we can give you is to commit to this practice, remain curious, continue to learn, let this process unfold, and watch it slowly begin to find its way into your daily life.

References

American Psychiatric Association. 2000. *Diagnostic and Statistical Manual of Mental Disorders: DSM-IV-TR.* 4th ed. Text rev. Arlington, VA: American Psychiatric Publishing.

Azari, N. P., J. Nickel, G. Wunderlich, M. Niedeggen, H. Hefter, L. Tellmann, H. Herzog, P. Stoerig, D. Birnbacher, and R. J. Seitz. 2001. "Neural Correlates of Religious Experience." *European Journal of Neuroscience* 13 (8):1649–52.

Azeemi, K. S. 2005. *Muraqaba: The Art and Science of Sufi Meditation.* Translated by S. S. Reaz. Houston, TX: Plato Publishing.

Barnard, L. K., and J. F. Curry. 2011. "Self-Compassion: Conceptualizations, Correlates, and Interventions." *Review of General Psychology* 15 (4):289–303.

Barnes, P. M., B. Bloom, and R. L. Nahin. 2008. "Complementary and Alternative Medicine Use among Adults and Children: United States, 2007." *National Health Statistics Reports* 12:1–23.

Bjorklund, P. 2006. "No Man's Land: Gender Bias and Social Constructivism in the Diagnosis of Borderline Personality Disorder." *Issues in Mental Health Nursing* 27 (1):3–23.

Black, D. W., N. Blum, B. Pfohl, and N. Hale. 2004. "Suicidal Behavior in Borderline Personality Disorder: Prevalence, Risk Factors, Prediction, and Prevention." *Journal of Personality Disorders* 18:226–39.

Bohus, M., M. Limberger, U. Ebner, F. X. Glocker, B. Schwarz, M. Wernz, and K. Lieb. 2000. "Pain Perception during Self-Reported Distress and Calmness in Patients with Borderline Personality Disorder and Self-Mutilating Behavior." *Psychiatry Research* 95:251–60.

Brefczynski-Lewis, J. A., A. Lutz, H. S. Schaefer, D. B. Levinson, and R. J. Davidson. 2007. "Neural Correlates of Attentional Expertise in Long-Term Meditation Practitioners." *Proceedings of the National Academy of Sciences* 104 (27):11483–88.

Brown, K. W., and R. M. Ryan. 2003. "The Benefits of Being Present: Mindfulness and Its Role in Psychological Well-Being." *Journal of Personality and Social Psychology* 84 (4):822–48.

Carlson, L. E., M. Speca, K. D. Patel, and E. Goodey. 2004. "Mindfulness-Based Stress Reduction in Relation to Quality of Life, Mood, Symptoms of Stress, and Levels of Cortisol, Dehydroepiandrosterone Sulfate (DHEAS), and Melatonin in Breast and Prostate Cancer Outpatients." *Psychoneuroendocrin-ology* 29 (4):448–74.

Carmody, J., and R. A. Baer. 2008. "Relationships between Mindfulness Practice and Levels of Mindfulness, Medical and Psychological Symptoms, and Well-Being in a Mindfulness-Based Stress Reduction Program." *Journal of Behavioral Medicine* 31 (1):23–33.

Chadwick, P., S. Hughes, D. Russell, I. Russell, and D. Dagnan. 2009. "Mindfulness Groups for Distressing Voices and Paranoia: A Replication and Randomized Feasibility Trial." *Behavioural and Cognitive Psychotherapy* 37 (4):403–12.

Chapman, A. L., K. L. Gratz, and M. Z. Brown. 2006. "Solving the Puzzle of Deliberate Self-Harm: The Experiential Avoidance Model." *Behaviour Research and Therapy* 44 (3):371–94.

Coccaro, E. F., C. S. Bergeman, and G. E. McClearn. 1993. "Heritability of Irritable Impulsiveness: A Study of Twins Reared Together and Apart." *Psychiatry Research* 48 (3):229–42.

Cohen, D. L., N. Wintering, V. Tolles, R. R. Townsend, J. T. Farrar, M. L. Galantino, and A. B. Newberg. 2009. "Cerebral Blood Flow Effects of Yoga Training: Preliminary Evaluation of 4 Cases." *Journal of Alternative and Complementary Medicine* 15 (1):9–14.

Cooper, J., N. Kapur, R. Webb, M. Lawlor, E. Guthrie, K. Mackway-Jones, and L. Appleby. 2005. "Suicide after Deliberate Self-Harm: A 4-Year Cohort Study." *American Journal of Psychiatry* 162 (2):297–303.

Corby, J. C., W. T. Roth, V. P Zarcone Jr., and B. S. Kopell. 1978. "Psychophysiological Correlates of the Practice of Tantric Yoga Meditation." *Archives of General Psychiatry* 35 (5):571–77.

Dorn, S. D., O. S. Palsson, S. I. M. Thiwan, M. Kanazawa, W. C. Clark, M. A. L. van Tilburg, D. A. Drossman, Y. Scarlett, R. L. Levy, Y. Ringel, M. D. Crowell, K. W. Olden, and W. E. Whitehead. 2007. "Increased Colonic Pain Sensitivity in Irritable Bowel Syndrome Is the Result of an Increased Tendency to Report Pain rather than Increased Neurosensory Sensitivity." *Gut* 56:1202–09.

Dutton, D. G., A. Starzomski, and L. Ryan. 1996. "Antecedents of Abusive Personality and Abusive Behavior in Wife Assaulters." *Journal of Family Violence* 11 (2):113–32.

Elson, B. D., P. Hauri, and D. Cunis. 1977. "Physiological Changes in Yoga Meditation." *Psychophysiology* 14 (1):52–57.

Finucane, A., and S. W. Mercer. 2006. "An Exploratory Mixed Methods Study of the Acceptability and Effectiveness of Mindfulness-Based Cognitive Therapy for Patients with Active Depression and Anxiety in Primary Care." *BMC Psychiatry* 6 (1):14.

Fertuck, E. A., A. Jekal, I. Song, B. Wyman, M. C. Morris, S. T. Wilson, B. S Brodsky, and B. Stanley. 2009. "Enhanced 'Reading the Mind in the Eyes' in Borderline Personality Disorder Compared to Healthy Controls." *Psychological Medicine* 39 (12):1979–88.

Forgas, J. P. 1999. "Feeling and Speaking: Mood Effects on Verbal Communication Strategies." *Personality and Social Psychology Bulletin* 25 (7):850–63.

Frankenburg, F. R., and M. C. Zanarini. 2004. "The Association between Borderline Personality Disorder and Chronic Medical Illnesses, Poor Health-Related Lifestyle Choices, and Costly Forms of Health Care Utilization." *Journal of Clinical Psychiatry* 65 (12):1660–65.

Fronsdal, G., trans. 2005. *The Dhammapada: A New Translation of the Buddhist Classic with Annotations*. 1st ed. Boston: Shambhala Publications.

Germer, C. K. 2009. *The Mindful Path to Self-Compassion: Freeing Yourself from Destructive Thoughts and Emotions*. New York: The Guilford Press.

Giacalone, R. C. 1997. "A Study of Clinicians' Attitudes and Sex Bias in the Diagnosis of Borderline Personality Disorder and Post-traumatic Stress Disorder." *Dissertation Abstracts International* 57:7725B.

Goodman, M., and A. New. 2000. "Impulsive Aggression in Borderline Personality Disorder." *Current Psychiatry Reports* 2 (1):56–61.

Goyer, P. F., P. J. Andreason, W. E. Semple, A. H. Clayton, A. C. King, B. A. Compton-Toth, S. C. Schulz, and R. M. Cohen. 1994. "Positron-Emission Tomography and Personality Disorders." *Neuropsychopharmacology* 10 (1):21–28.

Grant, B. F., S. P. Chou, R. B. Goldstein, B. Huang, F. S. Stinson, T. D. Saha, S. M. Smith, D. A. Dawson, A. J. Pulay, R. P. Pickering, and W. J. Ruan. 2008. "Prevalence, Correlates, Disability, and Comorbidity of *DSM-IV* Borderline Personality Disorder: Results from the Wave 2 National Epidemiologic Survey on Alcohol and Related Conditions." *Journal of Clinical Psychiatry* 69 (4):533–45.

Grilo, C. M., T. H McGlashan, L. C. Morey, J. G. Gunderson, A. E. Skodol, M. T. Shea, C. A. Sanislow, M. C. Zanarini, D. Bender, J. M. Oldham, I. Dyck, and R. L.Stout. 2001. "Internal Consistency, Intercriterion Overlap, and Diagnostic Efficiency of Criteria Sets for *DSM-IV* Schizotypal, Borderline, Avoidant, and Obsessive-Compulsive Personality Disorders. *Acta Psychiatrica Scandinavica* 104 (4):264–72.

Gunaratana, B. H. 2002. *Mindfulness in Plain English*. Somerville, MA: Wisdom Publications.

Hofmann, S. G., A. T. Sawyer, A. A. Witt, and D. Oh. 2010. "The Effect of Mindfulness-Based Therapy on Anxiety and Depression: A Meta-analytic Review." *Journal of Consultation Clinical Psychology* 78 (2):169–83.

Hollander, M. 2008. *Helping Teens Who Cut: Understanding and Ending Self-Injury*. New York: The Guilford Press.

Hölzel, B. K., U. Ott, H. Hempel, A. Hackl, K. Wolf, R. Stark, and D. Vaitl. 2007. "Differential Engagement of Anterior Cingulate and Adjacent Medial Frontal Cortex in Adept Meditators and Non-meditators." *Neuroscience Letters* 421 (1):16–21.

Kabat-Zinn, J. 1982. "An Outpatient Program in Behavioral Medicine for Chronic Pain Patients Based on the Practice of Mindful Meditation: Theoretical Considerations and Preliminary Results." *General Hospital Psychiatry* 4 (1):33–47.

————. 1994. *Wherever You Go, There You Are: Mindfulness Meditation in Everyday Life*. 1st ed. New York: Hyperion.

Kabat-Zinn, J., L. Lipworth, and R. Burney. 1985. "The Clinical Use of Mindfulness Meditation for the Self-Regulation of Chronic Pain." *Journal of Behavioral Medicine* 8 (2):163–90.

Kabat-Zinn, J., A. O. Massion, J. Kristeller, L. G. Peterson, K. E. Fletcher, L. Pbert, W. R. Lenderking, and S. F. Santorelli. 1992. "Effectiveness of a Meditation-Based Stress Reduction Program in the Treatment of Anxiety Disorders." *American Journal of Psychiatry* 149 (7):936–43.

Kimbrough, E., T. Magyari, P. Langenberg, M. Chesney, and B. Berman. 2010. "Mindfulness Intervention for Child Abuse Survivors." *Journal of Clinical Psychology* 66 (1):17–33.

Klonsky, E. D. 2008. "What Is Emptiness? Clarifying the 7th Criterion for Borderline Personality Disorder." *Journal of Personality Disorders* 22 (4):418–26.

Kreisman, J. J., and H. Straus. 1989. *I Hate You—Don't Leave Me: Understanding the Borderline Personality*. New York: Avon Books.

Kristeller, J. L., and C. B. Hallett. 1999. "An Exploratory Study of a Meditation-Based Intervention for Binge Eating Disorder." *Journal of Health Psychology* 4 (3):357–63.

Kubota, Y., W. Sato, M. Toichi, T. Murai, T. Okada, A. Hayashi, and A. Sengoku. 2001. "Frontal Midline Theta Rhythm Is Correlated with Cardiac Autonomic Activities during the Performance of an Attention Demanding Meditation Procedure." *Brain Research: Cognitive Brain Research* 11 (2):281–87.

Leichsenring, F., E. Leibing, J. Kruse, A. S. New, and F. Leweke. 2011. "Borderline Personality Disorder." *Lancet* 377 (9759):74–84.

Lester, D., and J. Bean. 1992. "Attribution of Causes to Suicide." *Journal of Social Psychology* 132 (5):679–80.

Li, D., and L. He. 2007. "Meta-analysis Supports Association between Serotonin Transporter (5-HTT) and Suicidal Behavior." *Molecular Psychiatry* 12:47–54.

Lidberg, L., H. Belfrage, L. Bertilsson, M. M. Evenden, and M. Asberg. 2000. "Suicide Attempts and Impulse Control Disorder Are Related to Low Cerebrospinal Fluid 5-HIAA in Mentally Disordered Violent Offenders." *Acta Psychiatrica Scandinavica* 101 (5):395–402.

Linehan, M. M. 1993. *Cognitive-Behavioral Treatment of Borderline Personality Disorder*. New York: The Guilford Press.

Ma, S. H., and J. D. Teasdale. 2004. "Mindfulness-Based Cognitive Therapy for Depression: Replication and Exploration of Differential Relapse Prevention Effects." *Journal of Consulting and Clinical Psychology* 72 (1):31–40.

Merton, T. 1960. *Spiritual Direction and Meditation*. Collegeville, MN: The Order of St. Benedict.

Michaelson, J. 2007. *God in Your Body: Kabbalah, Mindfulness, and Embodied Spiritual Practice*. Woodstock, VT: Jewish Lights Publishing.

Miller, J. J., K. Fletcher, and J. Kabat-Zinn. 1995. "Three-Year Follow-Up and Clinical Implications of a Mindfulness Meditation–Based Stress Reduction Intervention in the Treatment of Anxiety Disorders." *General Hospital Psychiatry* 17 (3):192–200.

Mruk, C. J. 2003. *Zen and Psychotherapy: Integrating Traditional and Nontraditional Approaches*. With J. Hartzell. New York: Springer Publishing Company.

Murata, T., T. Takahashi, T. Hamada, M. Omori, H. Kosaka, H. Yoshida, and Y. Wada. 2004. "Individual Trait Anxiety Levels Characterizing the Properties of Zen Meditation." *Neuropsychobiology* 50 (2):189–94.

Neff, K. D. 2003. "The Development and Validation of a Scale to Measure Self-Compassion." *Self and Identity* 2 (3):223–50.

New, A. S., R. L. Trestman, V. Mitropoulou, D. S. Benishay, E. Coccaro, J. Silverman, and L. J. Siever. 1997. "Serotonergic Function and Self-Injurious Behavior in Personality Disorder Patients." *Psychiatry Research* 69 (1):17–26.

Newberg, A., A. Alavi, M. Baime, M. Pourdehnad, J. Santanna, and E. d'Aquili. 2001. "The Measurement of Regional Cerebral Blood Flow during the Complex Cognitive Task of Meditation: A Preliminary SPECT Study." *Psychiatry Research* 106 (2):113–22.

Newberg, A. B., and J. Iversen. 2003. "The Neural Basis of the Complex Mental Task of Meditation: Neurotransmitter and Neurochemical Considerations." *Medical Hypotheses* 61 (2):282–91.

Nock, M. K. 2010. "Self-Injury." *Annual Review of Clinical Psychology* 6:339–63.

Perreau-Linck, E., M. Beauregard, P. Gravel, V. Paquette, J.-P. Soucy, M. Diksic, and C. Benkelfat. 2007. "In Vivo Measurements of Brain Trapping of 11C-Labelled β-Methyl-L-Tryptophan during Acute Changes in Mood States." *Journal of Psychiatry and Neuroscience* 32 (6):430–34.

Rosen, C. 2008. "The Myth of Multitasking." *New Atlantis* 20 (spring):105–10.

Ross, C. A. 2007. "Borderline Personality Disorder and Dissociation." *Journal of Trauma and Dissociation* 8 (1):71–80.

Russell, J. J., D. S. Moskowitz, D. C. Zuroff, D. Sookman, and J. Paris. 2007. "Stability and Variability of Affective Experience and Interpersonal Behavior in Borderline Personality Disorder." *Journal of Abnormal Psychology* 116 (3):578–88.

Salzberg, S. 2008. *Lovingkindness: The Revolutionary Art of Happiness*. Boston: Shambhala Publications.

———. 2010. *The Force of Kindness: Change Your Life with Love and Compassion*. Boulder, CO: Sounds True.

Sauer, S. E., and R. A. Baer. 2011. "Ruminative and Mindful Self-Focused Attention in Borderline Personality Disorder." *Personality Disorders: Theory, Research, and Treatment*, Epub ahead of print. doi:10.1037/a0025465.

Schnyder, U., L. Valach, K. Bichsel, and K. Michel. 1999. "Attempted Suicide: Do We Understand Patients' Reasons?" *General Hospital Psychiatry* 21 (1):62–69.

Schwartz, J. M., and S. Begley. 2002. *The Mind and the Brain: Neuroplasticity and the Power of Mental Force*. New York: ReganBooks.

Segal, Z. V., J. M. G. Williams, and J. D. Teasdale. 2002. *Mindfulness-Based Cognitive Therapy for Depression: A New Approach to Preventing Relapse.* New York: The Guilford Press.

Selby, E. A., T. W. Bender, K. H. Gordon, M. K. Nock, and T. E. Joiner Jr. 2012. "Non-Suicidal Self-Injury (NSSI) Disorder: A Preliminary Study." *Personality Disorders: Theory, Research, and Treatment* 3 (2):167–75.

Shearer, S. L. 1994. "Dissociative Phenomena in Women with Borderline Personality Disorder." *American Journal of Psychiatry* 151 (9):1324–28.

Simeon, D., D. Nelson, R. Elias, J. Greenberg, and E. Hollander. 2003. "Relationship of Personality to Dissociation and Childhood Trauma in Borderline Personality Disorder." *CNS Spectrums* 8 (10):755–62.

Simeon, D., B. Stanley, A. Frances, J. J. Mann, R. Winchel, and M. Stanley. 1992. "Self-Mutilation in Personality Disorders: Psychological and Biological Correlates." *American Journal of Psychiatry* 149 (2):221–26.

Smalley, S. L. 2010. "Mind Body Medicine: Can What You Think and Feel Affect Your Physical Health?" *Huffington Post*, The Blog, October 27. Retrieved May 30, 2012, from http.huffingtonpost.com/susan-smalley /how-whats-in-your-mind-ef_b_772813.html.

Soler, J., A. Valdepérez, A. Feliu-Soler, J. C. Pascual, M. J. Portella, A. Martín-Blanco, E. Alvarez, and V. Pérez. 2012. "Effects of the Dialectical Behavioral Therapy–Mindfulness Module on Attention in Patients with Borderline Personality Disorder." *Behaviour Research and Therapy* 50 (2):150–57.

Soloff, P. H., P. Pruitt, M. Sharma, J. Radwan, R. White, and V. A. Diwadkar. 2012. "Structural Brain Abnormalities and Suicidal Behavior in Borderline Personality Disorder." *Journal of Psychiatric Research* 46 (4):516–25.

Spoont, M. R. 1992. "Modulatory Role of Serotonin in the Neural Information Processing: Implications for Human Psychopathology." *Psychological Bulletin* 112 (2):330–50.

Stanley, B., L. Sher, S. Wilson, R. Ekman, Y. Y. Huang, and J. J. Mann. 2010. "Non-Suicidal Self-Injurious Behavior, Endogenous Opioids, and Monoamine Neurotransmitters." *Journal of Affective Disorders* 124 (1–2):134–40.

Stiglmayr, C. E., U. W. Ebner-Priemer, J. Bretz, R. Behm, M. Mohse, C.-H. Lammers, I.-G. Anghelescu, C. Schmahl, W. Schlotz, N. Kleindienst, and M. Bohus. 2008. "Dissociative Symptoms Are Positively Related to Stress in Borderline Personality Disorder." *Acta Psychiatrica Scandinavica* 117 (2):139–47.

Strong, M. 1998. "A Bright Red Scream: Self-Mutilation and the Language of Pain." New York: Viking.

Sudsuang, R., V. Chentanez, and K. Veluvan. 1991. "Effect of Buddhist Meditation on Serum Cortisol and Total Protein Levels, Blood Pressure, Pulse Rate, Lung Volume, and Reaction Time." *Physiology and Behavior* 50 (3):543–48.

Takahashi, T., T. Murata, T. Hamada, M. Omori, H. Kosaka, M. Kikuchi, H. Yoshida, and Y. Wada. 2005. "Changes in EEG and Autonomic Nervous

Activity during Meditation and Their Association with Personality Traits." *International Journal of Psychophysiology* 55 (2):199–207.

Tang, Y. Y., Y. Ma, J. Wang, Y. Fan, S. Feng, Q. Lu, Q. Yu, D. Sui, M. K. Rothbart, M. Fan, and M. I. Posner. 2007. "Short-Term Meditation Training Improves Attention and Self-Regulation." *Proceedings of the National Academy of Sciences* 104 (43):17152–56.

Teasdale, J. D., Z. V. Segal, J. M. G. Williams, V. A. Ridgeway, J. M. Soulsby, and M. A. Lau. 2000. "Prevention of Relapse/Recurrence in Major Depression by Mindfulness-Based Cognitive Therapy." *Journal of Consulting and Clinical Psychology* 68 (4):615–23.

Thích Nhât Hạnh. 1995. *Living Buddha, Living Christ.* Introduction by E. Pagels. Foreword by D. Steindl-Rast. New York: Riverhead Books.

Tragesser, S. L., D. Bruns, and J. M. Disorbio. 2010. "Borderline Personality Disorder Features and Pain: The Mediating Role of Negative Affect in a Pain Patient Sample." *Clinical Journal of Pain* 26 (4):348–53.

Torgersen, S. 2000. "Genetics of Patients with Borderline Personality Disorder." *Psychiatric Clinics of North America* 23 (1):1–9.

Tsering, G. T. 2005. *The Four Noble Truths: The Foundation of Buddhist Thought.* Somerville, MA: Wisdom Publications.

Virkkunen, M., M. Eggert, R. Rawlings, and M. Linnoila. 1996. "A Prospective Follow-Up Study of Alcoholic Violent Offenders and Fire Setters." *Archives of General Psychiatry* 53 (6):523–29.

Wallace, R. K., H. Benson, and A. F. Wilson. 1971. "A Wakeful Hypometabolic Physiologic State." *American Journal of Physiology* 221 (3):795–99.

Wilkinson-Ryan, A. B., and D. Westen. 2000. "Identity Disturbance in Borderline Personality Disorder: An Empirical Investigation." *American Journal of Psychiatry* 157 (4):528–41.

Wingenfeld, K., M. Driessen, B. Adam, and A. Hill. 2007. "Overnight Urinary Cortisol Release in Women with Borderline Personality Disorder Depends on Comorbid PTSD and Depressive Psychopathology." *European Psychiatry* 22 (5):309–12.

Zanarini, M. C., T. F. Ruser, F. R. Frankenburg, J. Hennen, and J. G. Gunderson. 2000. "Risk Factors Associated with the Dissociative Experiences of Borderline Patients." *Journal of Nervous and Mental Disease* 188 (1):26–30.

Zeidan, F., K. T. Martucci, R. A. Kraft, N. S. Gordon, J. G. McHaffie, and R. C. Coghill. 2011. "Brain Mechanisms Supporting the Modulation of Pain by Mindfulness Meditation." *Journal of Neuroscience* 31 (14):5540–48.

Zylowska, L., D. L. Ackerman, M. H. Yang, J. L. Futrell, N. L. Horton, T. S. Hale, C. Pataki, and S. L. Smalley. 2008. "Mindfulness Meditation Training in Adults and Adolescents with ADHD: A Feasibility Study." *Journal of Attention Disorders* 11 (6):737–46.

Blaise Aguirre, MD, is an assistant professor of psychiatry at Harvard Medical School. He is expert in child, adolescent, and adult psychotherapy, including dialectical behavior therapy (DBT) and psychopharmacology. He is the medical director of 3East at Harvard-affiliated McLean Hospital. Aguirre has been a staff psychiatrist at McLean since 2000 and is widely recognized for his extensive work in the treatment of mood and personality disorders in adolescents. He is the author of *Parenting Your Child with Autism; Biographies of Disease: Depression; Borderline Personality Disorder in Adolescents;* and *Helping Your Troubled Teen.*

Gillian Galen, PsyD, is an instructor in psychology at Harvard Medical School. She is the assistant director of training and senior psychologist at 3East at the Harvard-affiliated McLean Hospital—a unique, residential DBT program for young women exhibiting self-endangering behaviors and borderline personality traits. She specializes in adolescent psychotherapy, including DBT. She has a particular interest in using mindfulness and yoga in the treatment of BPD and other psychiatric illnesses. Galen has been a registered yoga instructor since 2008.